Experimental Pharmacology

for

Undergraduate Students

Experimental Pharmacology
for
Undergraduate Students

Dr. GOBIND RAI GARG

Dr. SAURABH ARYA

Department of Pharmacology,
University College of Medical Sciences &
GTB Hospital, Delhi - 110 095

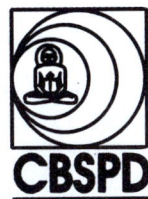

CBSPD

CBS Publishers & Distributors Pvt Ltd

New Delhi • Bengaluru • Chennai • Kochi • Kolkata • Lucknow • Mumbai
Hyderabad • Jharkhand • Nagpur • Patna • Pune • Uttarakhand

Experimental Pharmacology
for Undergraduate Students

ISBN: 978-81-239-1266-0

First Edition: 2005
Reprint: 2006, 2007, 2008, 2009, 2010, 2012, 2014, 2016, 2017, 2018, 2019, 2020, 2023, 2024

Published by **Satish Kumar Jain** and produced by **Varun Jain** for

CBS Publishers & Distributors Pvt Ltd

4819/XI Prahlad Street, 24 Ansari Road, Daryaganj, New Delhi 110 002, India.

Ph: 011-23289259, 23266861

Website: www.cbspd.com
e-mail: delhi@cbspd.com

Corporate Office: 204 FIE, Industrial Area, Patparganj, Delhi 110 092

Ph: 011-4934 4934

Fax: 011-4934 4935   e-mail: publishing@cbspd.com;publicity@cbspd.com

Branches

- **Bengaluru:** Seema House 2975, 17th Cross, K.R. Road, Banasankari 2nd Stage, Bengaluru 560 070, Karnataka, India
  Ph: +91-80-26771678/79   Fax: +91-80-26771680   e-mail: bangalore@cbspd.com
- **Chennai:** 7, Subbaraya Street, Shenoy Nagar, Chennai 600 030, Tamil Nadu, India
  Ph: +91-44-26680620, 26681266   Fax: +91-44-42032115   e-mail: chennai@cbspd.com
- **Kochi:** 42/1325, 1326, Power House Road, Opp KSEB, Ernakulam 682 018, Kochi, Kerala, India
  Ph: +91-484-4059061-67   Fax: +91-484-4059065   e-mail: kochi@cbspd.com
- **Kolkata:** 147, Hind Ceramics Compound, 1st Floor, Nilgunj Road, Belghoria, Kolkata 700 056, West Bengal, India
  Ph: +91-33-25633055/56   e-mail: kolkata@cbspd.com
- **Lucknow:** Basement, Khushnuma Complex, 7-Meerabai Marg (Behind Jawahar Bhawan), Lucknow 226 001, UP, India
  Ph: +0552-4000032   e-mail:tiwari.lucknowi@cbspd.com
- **Mumbai:** PWD Shed. Gala no. 25/26, Ramchandra Bhatt Marg, Next to JJ Hospital Gate no. 2, Opp. Union Bank of India, Noorbaug, Mumbai 400 009, Maharashtra, India
  Ph: 022-66661880/89   e-mail: mumbai@cbspd.com

Representatives

| Hyderabad | 0-9885175004 | Jharkhand | 0-9811541605 | Nagpur | 0-8692091830 |
| Patna | 0-9334159340 | Pune | 0-9664372571 | Uttarakhand | 0-9716462459 |

Printed at: SRK Graphics, Shahdara, Delhi

Dedicated to
our beloved parents,
family members,
Monica Arya &
Praveen Goswami

PREFACE

Discovery consists of seeing what everybody has seen
and thinking what nobody has thought.
— **Albert Gyorgyi**

From our experience as teachers, we felt the need of a book on experimental pharmacology for undergraduate students. This book contains the basic principle of each experiment included in the curriculum as well as all the details. Most importantly, viva questions for each experiment have been given at the end of each experiment. We have seen that students fumble at the oral table even when asked the easiest of questions. This occurs inspite of having studied everything several times. This is because they fail to assimilate the important bits of information at the time of examinations. This effort of ours underlines the important aspects of experimental pharmacology in very simple language to help students retain more.

We are grateful to Dr. K.K. Sharma, Professor and Head, Department of Pharmacology, University College of Medical Sciences, Delhi; and other teachers of our department; Dr. P. Mahajan, Dr. S.K. Bhattacharya, Dr. P.K. Mediratta and Dr. N. Khanna, whose guidance in our postgraduate training has brought us to the stage of writing this practical book with so much confidence.

We are especially thankful to **DR. DEEPIKA ARORA**, ex-senior demonstrator, Department of Pharmacology, UCMS, without whose help this work would not even have started. We are also thankful to all our colleagues for their continuous encouragement.

Our sincere gratitude is due, to Shri B.M. Singh (Production Incharge) and Shri R.K. Saxena (Pagitek Graphics, Delhi), for their painstaking and creative efforts in bringing out this book.

At last and above all we are grateful to our parents and family members for their emotional support, encouragement and valuable co-operation even in our hard days while authoring the book.

Dr. Gobind Rai Garg
&
Dr. Saurabh Arya
PG, Dept. of Pharmacology
UCMS & GTB Hospital
Delhi-110095

CONTENTS

PART-III

AMPHIBIAN EXPERIMENTS

PART-IV

PRESCRIPTION WRITING

PART-V

CLINICAL CASES

PART-VI

COMMENTS

PART-I
Pharmacy Practical

1. GENERAL

In this part of the examination, a preparation has to be made and viva-voce will be taken. The following things are required to be done in the pharmacy practical.

1. Make the preparation
2. Paste the label on it
3. Content to be written on answer sheet
4. Write the prescription
5. Viva Voce.

Pharmacy practical consists of 5 marks and for every preparation, prescription and labelling has to be done.

1. **Prescription:** It is a very important part of the pharmacy practical. Also a separate question carrying 5 marks is given asking for the prescription of a particular disease. So it is very scoring.

Definition of Prescription: A prescription is a written order by a doctor to a pharmacist to supply certain medicinal substances in a particular form to a patient, to be used as directed.

1. MAKING THE PREPARATION

For making the preparation, the following are the necessary requirements:

(i) All the ingredients and their concentrations must be known.

(ii) The correct apparatus must be used.

(iii) Small scissors, scale and fractional weights must be brought to the examination by the students.

(iv) Each preparation should be dispensed in the correct apparatus.

(v) Correct cap (if required) should be tied with the pharmaceutical knot.

(vi) Proper labelling should be done.

(vii) After completing the exercise, all apparatus used should be washed and returned.

FORMAT OF A PRESCRIPTION

(i) Doctor's particulars should be written on the upper right hand corner. The name should be written in full and not as XYZ/ABC etc. Address must also be mentioned. Date should be written below, the doctors address.

(ii) Patients particulars must be written on the left hand corner below the doctor's particulars. Here also name, age, sex and registration no. must be mentioned.

(iii) Diagnosis has to be written below the patients particulars.

(iv) Parts of prescription. (Refer to model prescription on page 5)

(a) *Superscription:* This is the symbol R_j. It means 'take thou' i.e. you take. It is to be written as '℞' not 'R_x'. 'R' means Recipe and 'J' is an invocation to Jupiter, the god of healing, learning and knowledge.

(b) *Inscription:* It is the body of the prescription and consists of the name of ingredients and the quantities of each ingredient.

Traditionally, the inscription is divided into 4 parts.

(i) *Basis:* It is the principal drug and is responsible for the main action of the prescription.

(ii) *Adjuvant:* It increases the action of the basis.

(iii) *Corrective:* Corrects the undesirable effects of basis/adjuvant.

(iv) *Vehicle:* It is the agent used as solvent in the preparation.

(c) *Subscription:* Direction to pharmacist.

(d) *Signa:* Directions to patient. (Not the signature of the doctor).

(e) *Initials:* Signature of doctor with Regd. no.

* **Note:** Prescription is an order for the pharmacist and not for the patient.

S.No.	Preparation	Apparatus	Dispensed in	Cap	Secondary label	Precaution
1.	Condy's Lotion	Glass Mortar and Pestle	Colored bottle	Red	Upper only	Wax paper should be put on cork.
2.	Calamine Lotion	Glass Mortar and Pestle	Dispensing bottle	Red	Both upper and lower	–
3.	Siedlitz Powder	Porcelain mortar and pestle	2 inner and 1 outer packet	None	None	–
4.	Mandl's Paint	Glass mortar and pestle	Wide mouthed bottle	Red	Both upper and lower	Wax paper should be put on cork
5.	Tincture Iodine	Glass mortar and pestle	Colored bottle	Red	Upper only	Wax paper should be put on cork
6.	Liniment Turpentine	Porcelain mortar and pestle	Colored bottle	Red	Upper & lower	Wax paper should be put on cork.
7.	Carminative Mixture	Glass mortar and pestle	Dispensing bottle	White	None	Dose label must be put.
8.	Whitfield's Ointment	Porcelain tile, spatula and china dish	Pill Box	None	Upper only	Secondary label should be semicircular
9.	Benzyl Benzoate Emulsion	Porcelain mortar and pestle	Wide mouthed bottle	None	Upper and lower both	Mix in one direction only
10.	ORS	Tile and spatula	Outer and inner packet	None	None	–
11.	Hyoscine Hydrobromide Powder	Tile & Spatula	Outer & inner packet	None	None	–
12.	APC powder	Tile & Spatula	Outer & inner packet	None	None	–
13.	Castor Oil Emulsion	Porcelain mortar and pestle	Dispensing Bottle	White	One (Lower only)	Mix in one direction only
14.	Shark Liver Emulsion	Porcelain mortar and pestle	Dispensing Bottle	White	Lower only	Mix in one direction only
15.	Sulphur Ointment	Porcelain Tile, spatula & china dish	Pill Box	None	Upper only	Secondary label should be semi-circular

MODEL OF A PRESCRIPTION

(i)
> Dr. Deepika, MD.
> H-27 Sec. 29. Noida.
> Regd. No. 23819

Date: 27-11-03

(ii)
> Patient's Name: Sohan Lal
> Age/Sex: 25/M
> Reg. No. 2225

(iii)
> Δ - Amoebiasis

(iv) (a)
> ℞

(b)
> Tab Metronidazole 400mg tds × 5 days

(c)
> Send such 15 tablets.

(d)
> Take 1 tablet three times a day for 5 days.

(e)
> *Deepika*
> Regd. No 23819.

2. LABELLING

After preparing the prescription a label has to be pasted on the dispensing apparatus. The following points must be kept in mind while preparing the label:

1. It should be neat and clean.
2. It should be neatly cut with the help of scissors.
3. It consists of two parts, primary and secondary. Primary label should include the preparation.
4. Particulars of the patient, direction to the patient, place of preparation and the signature of the pharmacist must be included in the label. Particulars of the patient must have same name like Sudhir Kumar and not ABC.
5. Width of primary and secondary label should be equal.
6. There should be a small gap between primary and secondary labels.
7. The combined length of both the labels should be equal to 2/3rds of the length of the bottle.
8. Equal gap should be left on upper and lower margin.
9. Label should be put on the dispensing bottle on the side opposite to that containing dose markings i.e. smooth surface, and it should cover three surfaces of the dispensing bottle.
10. In case of colored bottle, the label should cover half the circumference of the bottle.

MODEL OF LABELS FOR BENZYL BENZOATE EMULSION

FOR EXTERNAL USE ONLY

Secondary Label

THE EMULSION

Name : Sudhir Kumar

Age : 12 years

Sex : Male

Regd. No. : 3162.

Directions: Apply all over the body below neck after a hot scrubbed bath. Repeat application after 12 hours followed by a bath, with change of clothings.

UCMS Pharmacy
21-11-2003

Sanjay
(Pharmacist)

Primary Label

SHAKE WELL BEFORE USE

Secondary Label

3. CONTENT TO BE WRITTEN ON ANSWER SHEET

1. Aim
2. Apparatus required
3. Composition
4. Procedure is brief
5. Prescription
6. Uses of Preparation
7. Uses of ingredients
8. Precautions

4. VIVA-VOCE

These are some general questions that can be asked in the viva-voce. Specific viva questions for each preparation are given along with each preparation ahead.

Q. 1. What is a drug?

Ans. A drug is a substance or product that is used to modify or explore physiological systems or pathological states for the benefit of the recipient.

Q. 2. What is pharmacy?

Ans. It is the science and act of compounding and dispensing drugs for the purpose of administration to the patient.

Q. 3. What is Pharmacognosy?

Ans. It is the science dealing with identification of drugs.

Q. 4. What is pharmacopoeia?

Ans. It is an official code containing a selected list of established drugs and medicinal preparations with description of their physical properties and lists their identity, purity and potency.

Q. 5. What is meant by I.P. and B.P.?

Ans. IP stands for Indian Pharmacopoeia & B.P. stands for British Pharmacopoeia.

Q. 6. What is meant by 1% solution?

Ans. It means 1 gm of solute is present in 100 ml of the solution.

Q. 7. What is meant by 1:1000 Acetyl choline solution?

Ans. It means 1 gm of acetylcholine is present in 1000 ml of the solution.

Q. 8. What are the various household measures used.

Ans. These are:

1. 1 Teaspoonful - 5 ml
2. 1 Table spoonful - 15 ml
3. 1 Dessert Spoonful - 8 ml
4. 1 Tea cup - 150 ml
5. 1 Glassful - 250 ml

Q. 9. What is meant by

a.c.	= ante cibum (before meals)
p.c.	= Post cibum (after meals)
a.d.	= adjust (upto)
ad.lib.	= ad libitum (at pleasure)
b.d.	= bis in die (twice a day)
t.d.s.	= ter in die (thrice a day)
q.i.d.	= quarter in die (four times a day)
h.s.	= horu somni (at bed time)
o.h.	= omni hora (every hour)
stat	= statum (immediately)
m	= misce (mix)
ft	= flat (make)
mit	= mitte (send)
s.o.s	= si opus sit (if necessary)

Q. 10. What are schedule H. drugs?

Ans. These are the drugs which must be sold by retail only when a prescription from a registered medical practitioner (RMP) is produced.

Q. 11. What are schedule G. drugs?

Ans. These are dangerous drugs on which a label of caution must be pasted and should be taken under medical supervision only.

Q. 12. What is a mixture?

Ans. It is a aqueous preparation of medicament which is meant for oral use only. It can be a solution or a suspension.

Solution: soluble substance in water.

Suspension: Insoluble substance in water.

Q. 13. What is the difference between lotion and solution?

Ans. Both are aqueous preparations of medicament. Lotion is for external use whereas solution is for oral use.

Q. 14. What is a gel?

Ans. It is a thick colloidal preparation in which drug particles are suspended eg. Aluminium hydroxide gel.

Q. 15. What is an Elixer?

Ans. It is a clear liquid preparation of medicament for oral use. It is made for drugs which cause nausea. It is prepared by adding flavouring agents to the drug.

Q. 16. What is Linctus?

Ans. These are viscous liquid preparations usually containing medicaments having local action on the mucus membrane of the throat. They are sipped slowly.

Q. 17. What are enteric coated tablets?

Ans. These are pills or tablets which are coated with keratin, shellac, or cellulose acid phosphate. These substances are not soluble in gastric juice but are dissolved by intestinal juices. These are used for the drugs which get destroyed by gastric acids.

Q. 18. Why is a red cap used in certain preparations?

Ans. Because it indicates "for external use only". It is put on preparations meant for external use.

Q. 19. Which preparations are dispensed in colored bottles?

Ans. Substances sensitive to light are dispensed in colored bottles.

NOTES

_____
_____
_____
_____
_____
_____
_____
_____
_____
_____
_____
_____
_____
_____
_____
_____
_____
_____

NOTES

2. SPECIFIC PHARMACY PREPARATIONS

1. Condy's Lotion (Potassium Permanganate solution 1: 1000)

Aim:

To prepare and dispense 20 ml of Condy's solution (1:1000 potassium permangenate)

Apparatus:

Balance, fractional weights, glass mortar and pestle, measuring cylinder of 100 ml capacity, coloured bottle, cork, cap, thread, white paper, wax paper, brown paper, scissors, spirit lamp, gum, shellac, distilled water.

Procedure:

100 mg of potassium permanganate crystals were weighed and ground finely in the glass mortar and pestle. 20 ml of water was added to it and mixed well. The fluid was then transferred to the measuring cylinder and water was added upto 100 ml.

20 ml of this solution was taken in the colored bottle and the mouth was closed with a cork coated with wax paper (to prevent staining and oxidation of the cork with $KMnO_4$). The cork should be of a suitable size and it should fit into the mouth of the bottle in such a way that 1/3 rd of its is inside the bottle and 2/3 is outside the bottle. A red coloured cap was put over the cork and a pharmaceutical knot was tied at the neck of the bottle: Labelling of the bottle is done as follows (copy from viva questions). The bottle was then wrapped with brown paper. The length of the paper should be 3″ more than the length of the bottle (1″ at the top and 2″ below). The width of the paper should be 3 times the width of the bottle. The paper was then folded into 2 parts such that one half is 1/2″ bigger than the other. The extra paper is then folded at that line. Now the brown paper was wrapped round the bottle so that the folded margin is exactly in the midline of the flat surface of the bottle. Then the 2 ends of the paper were folded and sealed by lae.

Viva Questions

Q. 1.   What is a Lotion?

Ans.   It is an aqueous suspension or solution meant for external use or local application.

Q. 2.   What is the difference between lotion and liniment?

1. Lotion has an aqueous vehicle whereas linement doesn't.
2. Lotion is applied without friction whereas friction is required for application of liniment.

Q. 3.   What are the uses of $KMnO_4$?

Ans.   (i)   As crystals - In snake bite

(ii)   As 1:1000 solution - for sterilization of instruments, washing of clothes worn by persons having infectious diseases.

(iii)   As 1:4000 solution - for vaginal and urethral irrigation.

(iv)   As 1:5000 solution- for gargles, mouth wash, gum diseases.

(v)   As 1:200 solution - for stomach wash in morphine, phosphorus, and strychnine poisoning.

(vi)   1:100 solution - for fungal infection.

Q. 4.   What is the mechanism of action of $KMnO_4$?

Ans. $KMnO_4$ acts as an oxidizing agent by liberating nascent oxygen which causes oxidation of microbes.

Q. 5.   Why is $KMnO_4$ used for stomach wash in case of morphine poisoning due to its I/V use?

Ans.   Morphine is actively secreted in the stomach and so it is oxidized by $KMnO_4$ and thus destroyed.

Q. 6.   Why is glass mortar and pestle used instead of porcelain mortar and pestle in preparing $KMnO_4$ soln.?

Ans. $KMnO_4$ reacts with porcelain and also stains it, so glass mortar and pestle is used.

Q. 7.   Why do you wrap the cork with wax paper?

Ans. Because cork should not be allowed to come in contact with $KMnO_4$ as it will get oxidized.

Q. 8. Name the other lotion that is prepared in your laboratory?

Ans. Calamine lotion.

Q. 9. Name the various preparations for which glass mortar & pestle should be used:

Ans. 1. Condy's Lotion
2. Calamine Lotion
3. Mandle's Paint
4. Tincture Iodine
5. Carminature Mixture.

Q. 10. Name the preparations for which porcelain mortar & pestle can be used.

1. Siedlitz Powder
2. Liniment Turpentine
3. Whitfield Ointment
4. Benzyl Benzoate Emulsion.

Q. 11. Why is Condy's lotion diluted 5 times for gargling?

Ans. Because for gargling we need 1:5000 solution of $KMnO_4$ whereas Condy's lotion is the name for 1:1000 $KMnO_4$ solution.

Q. 12. Write the label for Condy's lotion (1:1000 $KMnO_4$).

FOR EXTERNAL USE ONLY

THE LOTION

Name   : Somta

Age   : 23 yrs

Sex   : Female

Reg. No. : 34621

Directions: Dilute 5 times and gargle twice a day in between meals.

UCMS Pharmacy   *Sunil*
8.12.03

13. Write the prescription for Condy's Lotion

Ans.

Dr. Saurabh Arya, MD
B-6, III, Sec-3, Rohini
Date: 10-12-03

Randheer Singh
30 yrs/Male
Regd. No. 3310

Δ Gingivitis

℞

Potassium Permagnate	20mg
Aqua Ad	20ml

Mix and make and send such 20 ml. solution.

Dilute 5 times and gargle twice a day in between meals.

Saurabh Arya
Regd No. 01/050

Q. 14. What is the solubility of $KMnO_4$?

Ans: 1 in 16 parts of water at 20°C.

Q. 15. What is an antiseptic?

Ans: It is a chemical substance which prevents the growth of microorganisms. It can be used safely on living tissues.

Q. 16. What is Rideal Walker (R.W.) coefficient?

Ans: R.W. coefficient is also known as phenol coefficient. The antiseptic or disinfectant property of a substance is compared by taking phenol as standard. It is calculated as:

$$\frac{\text{Maximum dilution of antiseptic/disinfectant that kills 24 hr old culture of Bacillus typhosis at 37° in 7-12 min}}{\text{Maximum dilution of phenol that kills the same culture in identical conditions}}$$

Q. 17. Name other oxidizing agents?

Ans. H_2O_2, Potassium perchlorate.

2. Calamine Lotion

Aim:

To prepare and dispense 50 ml of calamine lotion.

Apparatus:

Balance with fractional weights, glass mortar and pestle, dispensing bottle, measuring cylinder, cork, red paper, cap, thread, white paper, wax paper, brown paper, shellac, scissors, ruler, spirit lamp and chemicals.

Composition:

Ingredients for 50 ml

Calamine	7.5 gm
Zinc oxide	2.5 gm
Bentonite	1.5 gm
Glycerine	2.5 ml
Aqua ad	50 ml

Procedure:

The requisite amounts of calamine, zinc oxide and bentonite were weighed separately and ground together in mortar and pestle. 2.5 ml glycerine and 10 ml water were added to it and made into a fine paste. This was transferred into a measuring cylinder, the mortar and pestle were rinsed with a little more of the vehicle and transferred into the cylinder till the volume was made upto 50 ml. It was dispensed in a dispensing bottle, corked and a red cap was put. The pharmaceutical knot was tied. Labelling was done as follows. The bottle was then wrapped in brown paper and sealed.

Viva Questions

Q. 1. What is a lotion?

Ans. See previous pages.

Q. 2. What is difference between lotion & liniment.

Ans. See previous pages.

Q. 3. What are the various ingredients of calamine lotion

Ans.
Ingredients	Amount
Calamine	150g
ZnO	50g
Bentonite	30g
Glycerine	50g
Aqua Ad	1000ml

Q. 4. What are the uses of calamine lotion?

Ans. Eczema

Impetigo

Dermatitis

Sunburns

Itching

Varicose ulcers

Psoriasis

Q. 5. What is lacto calamine?

Ans: It is the market preparation of calamine lotion which contains casein and phenol also. Casein acts as a soothing agent and phenol acts as preservative and antiseptic.

Q. 6. What is the composition of calamine and give their uses?

Ans: Calamine is a natural ore having 98% ZnO and 2% Fe_2O_3.

ZnO acts as antiseptic, astringent and antipruritic.

Ferric oxide. Cosmetic value (gives pink colour).

Q. 7. Why is ZnO added in calamine lotion although calamine itself contains ZnO?

Ans. Calamine also contains ferric oxide which has an irritant action. To decrease the irritative action of calamine additional ZnO is used as it dilutes the ferric oxide.

Q. 8. What is bentonite and why is it used?

Ans. Bentonite is hydrated aluminium silicate. It has protective effect and helps to make the solution uniform.

Q. 9. Why is glycerine used?

Ans. It is hygroscopic (i.e. absorbs moisture). It prevents drying of the lotion. So, the preparation remains at the site of application for a longer time. It also functions as antiseptic and emolient.

Q. 10. What is an astringent?

Ans. It is a substance which precipitates proteins from the cells of the superficial layer and thereby forms a protective covering which prevents the action of irritants.

Q. 11. Give examples of some astringents.

Ans. Vegetable astringent – Tannic acid

Mineral astringent – Calamine

Q. 12. What is an emolient?

Ans. It is an agent which softens the skin by forming an occlusive oil film on the stratum corneum. It also prevents drying of the skin.

Q. 13. What will happen if calamine lotion is swallowed?

Ans. There will be vomiting because zinc irritates the stomach and also stimulates the CTZ.

Q. 14. Write the label for calamine lotion.

FOR EXTERNAL USE ONLY

THE LOTION

Name   : Mohit

Age   : 40 yrs

Sex   : Male

Regd. No : 1025

Directions : Apply on the affected part twice a day.

UCMS Pharmacy   *Sunil*
8-12-03

SHAKE THE BOTTLE BEFORE USE

Q. 15. Write the prescription of calamine lotion.

Dr. Gobind Garg
D-30, GTB Enclave
Regd. No.-2003/UCMS/225
Date: 8-12-03

Sandeep Singh
12 yr/Male
Regd. No. 3310

Δ Eczema
  ℞

Calamine	15g
ZnO	5g
Bentonite	3g
Glycerine	5g
Aqua Ad	100ml

Mix and make and send such 100ml.

Apply on the affected part thrice a day.

Gobind
Regd. No.-2003/UCMS/225

---

3. Siedlitz Powder

Aim:

To prepare and dispense a single dose of Siedlitz powder.

Apparatus:

Balance with weights, mortar and pestle, spatula, blue paper, white paper, chemicals.

Composition:

It consists of two powders packed separately

Powder A: Sodium potassium tartarate   7.5 gm
            Sodium bicarbonate   2.5 gm
Powder B: Tartaric acid   2.5 gm

Procedure:

7.5 gm of sodium potassium tartarate and 2.5 gm of sodium bicarbonate were weighed separately and mixed together and wrapped in blue paper (5″ × 7″) and marked as Powder A.

2.5 gm of Tartaric acid was then weighed separately, wrapped in wax paper (5″ × 7″) and marked as powder B.

The outer packing in white paper (7″ × 9″) was given as before.

Labelling was done.

Viva Questions

Q. 1   What is a powder?
Ans.   It is a preparation of medicament which is finely grounded.

Q. 2   What are the ingredients of Siedlitz powder?
Ans.   It consists of two powders.

Powder A - Na K Tartarate 7.5g ⎤ Packed in
            $NaHCO_3$ 2.5g ⎦ blue paper

Powder B - Tartaric Acid 2.5g ⎤ Packed in
                              ⎦ wax paper

Q. 3   Why is powder B wrapped in wax paper & not in colored paper?
Ans.   1. Tartaric acid is hygroscopic and it will absorb moisture and if wrapped in colored paper it will become soggy.
       2. Colored paper contains alkali. As tartaric acid is an acid, it will react with the alkali and lead to decolourisation of the paper.

Q. 4   How should this preparation be used and why?
Ans.   Powder A is mixed in water and then powder B is added. The solution is then drunk preferably early morning.
       If the powder is taken orally and then water is taken, a lot of CO_2 will be released suddenly according to the reaction given below.
       Tartaric acid + $NaHCO_3$ → Na Tartarate + CO_2
       This sudden release of CO_2 can lead to perforation of stomach. Powder A is added just because it is more bulky and takes longer time to dissolve and if it is added after Powder B, all the CO_2 will be dissolved.
       This powder is taken early morning because its onset of action is very short.

Q. 5   What are the uses of Siedlitz powder?
Ans.   It is used as a saline purgative in case of
       1. Constipation
       2. Along with antihelmenthics to expel worms.

Q. 6   After which antihelmenthic drug should Seidiltz powder be taken?
Ans.   It is taken after piperazine and niclosamide because it expels the dead worms (due to the paralysing action of piperazine and niclosamide). If the dead worms are allowed to remain in the intestine, they will secrete toxic fluid leading to fatal consequences.

Q. 7   Name a purgative which has a long onset of action.
Ans.   Bisacodyl (marked as Dulcolax) has a long onset of action. So it is given at night. It is used before radioactive procedures for emptying the stomach so that gases do not interfere with the radiographic results.
       It is used for - XRay KUB
       - Barium studies.

Q. 8   What is the advantage of the CO_2 that is produced?
Ans.   It masks the bitter taste of the salt and gives a pleasant sensation.

Q. 9   What is the mechanism of action of Siedlitz powder?
Ans.   Na K Tartarate and Na Tartarate are not absorbed from the intestine and thus causes softening of stools due to their osmotic action.

Q. 10 Write the label for Siedlitz powder.

THE POWDER

Name   :   Ranjit Arora

Age   :   25/M

Sex   :   Male

Regd. No. :   4410

Direction: Mix powder A in half glass of water, then add powder B, and drink while effervescent in early morning, empty stomach.

UCMS Pharmacy   *Rajat*
8.12.03

Q. 11 What is Rochelle's salt?

Ans. It is NaK Tartarate.

Q. 12 What are the other uses of $NaHCO_3$?

Ans. It is
 – Antacid
 – Carminative
 – Systemic alkalizer.

Q. 13 Why is it called Siedlitz powder?

Ans. It derived its name from a spring in West Germany, the water of which has purgative properties. (However the spring contains $MgSO_4$ and not NaK tartarate).

Q. 14 Name other saline purgatives.

Ans. Epsom Salt $(MgSO_4)$
 – Milk of Magnesia $(Mg(OH)_2)$
 – Glauber's Salt (Na_2SO_4)

Q. 15 Write the prescription for Seidlitz powder.

Dr. Tarun Arora
R. No. 444 GD Road,
C.P.
Regd. No. 2003/UCMS/01
Date: 8-03-2003

Mark Taylor
41/Male
Regd No. 3150

Δ. Constipation

℞

Powder A	NaK Tartarate	7.5 g
	$NaHCO_3$	2.5 g
Powder B	Tartaric Acid	2.5 g

Mix powder A in half glass of water, then add powder B and drink while effervescent in early morning, empty stomach.

Tarun
Regd. No. 2003/UCMS/01

---

4. Mandl's Paint

Aim:

To prepare and dispense 20 ml of Mandl's paint.

Apparatus:

Balance with fractional weights, glass mortar and pestle, wide mouthed reagent bottle with stopper, measuring cylinder, pippete, distilled water, white paper, brown paper, wax paper, scissors, shellac, gum, spirit lamp and chemicals.

Composition:

Ingredients	For 20 ml
Iodine	250 mg
Potassium Iodide	500 mg
Water	0.5 ml
Oil of peppermint	0.08 ml
Alcohol	0.75 ml
Glycerine ad	20 ml

Procedure:

500 mg of potassium iodide was taken in a glass mortar, powdered well and mixed with 0.5 ml of water. Then 250 mg of iodine was added and mixed with it. To this a small amount of glycerine was added to make a pigment. When all the iodine was completely dissolved the pigment was transferred to a measuring cylinder and to this 0.75 ml of alcohol and one drop of oil of peppermint was added. The mortar was rinsed with glycerine to produce the total volume upto 20 ml. A red paper cap and pharmaceutical knot were put. Labelling of the bottle was done.

Viva Questions

Q. 1 What is a paint?

Ans. It is a thick, viscid, syrupy preparation containing glycerine, meant for applying on mucus membrane.

Q. 2 What is the other name for Mandl's paint.

Ans. Pigmentrum sodi composita, also throat paint.

Q. 3 What is meant by Pigmentum?

Ans. Coloured.

Q. 4 What are the ingredients of Mandl's paint.

Ans.

Ingredients	For 100 ml	For 20 ml
I_2	1.25 ml	250 mg
KI	2.5 ml	500 mg
Water	2.5 ml	0.5 ml
Oil of peppermint	0.4 ml	0.08 ml
Alcohol	3.75 ml	0.75 ml
Glycerine ad	100 ml	20 ml

Q. 5 Tell the brief procedure.

Ans. KI was first powdered and wetted with water. To this I_2 was added and a small quantity of glycerine was added. When iodine was completely dissolved, alcohol and oil of peppermint was added. Glycerine was added to make volume of 20 ml. Red paper cap was tied with a pharmaceutical knot.

Q. 6 Why is KI first dissolved in water and then I_2 is added and not all three added together?

Ans. I_2 does not react with anhydrous potassium iodide. So KI is first mixed with water. Iodine then reacts with it to form nascent Iodine which is responsible for oxidation.

Q. 7 What are the functions of the various ingredients?

Ans.

1. Iodine – It acts as antiseptic as well as bactericidal. It reacts with KI to liberate nascent iodine,
   $$I_2 + KI \rightarrow KI_3 \rightarrow KI + 2 [I].$$
   Nascent iodine is responsible for oxidation. Its use is restricted to superficial parts only.

2. Oil of peppermint gives flavour. It has a mild antiseptic and cooling effect.

3. KI is used to dissolve I_2.

4. Alcohol has antiseptic action but is mainly used as a solvent for iodine.

5. Glycerine is hygroscopic in nature. It sticks to the surface of application and thus prolongs the action of iodine. Since glycerine has a sweet taste, it also makes the preparation palatable.

Q. 8 What are the uses of Mandl's paint?

Ans. Sore throat

Pharygitis

Tonsilitis

Q. 9 Why is glass mortar and pestle used?

Ans. Because iodine stains the porcelain mortar and pestle.

Q. 10 How is the paint applied?

Ans. It should be applied in the throat by a cotton swab twice a day in between meals.

Q. 11 Why is it applied in between meals and not before or after?

Ans. Because if applied before meals, it will be removed by the food, and if given just after meals, the tinkling of the throat may result in vomiting.

Q. 12 Which ingredient may be substituted?

Ans. Potassium iodide may be replaced with sodium iodide.

Q. 13 Name other preparations of iodine.

Ans.1. Liquid iodi fortis (strong solution of iodine)
→ 10% Iodine in 6% K1.

2. Liquid iodi mitis (Tincture Iodine)
→ 2% I_2 in 2.5% KI.

3. Lugol's iodine 5% I_2 in 10% KI →
It is used for preoperative preparation of a thyrotoxic patient to reduce the vascularity of the thyroid gland.

4. Non-staining iodine ointment- 5% I_2, used as fungicide.

5. I_2 is used as an ingredient in radioopaque contrast media.

6. Radioactive iodine (I^{131}) used for diagnosis and treatment of thyroid disorders.

Q. 14 Name other commonly used paints.

1. Boroglycerine paint – for stomatitis

2. Brilliant green and gentian violet - for non-exudative skin lesions.

3. Triple dye   Gentian violet

                      Brilliant green

                      Proflavine

4. Podophyllin compound paint - for warts

5. Tannic acid glycerine paint - to arrest bleeding from gums.

Q. 15 In which bottle should it be dispensed and why?

Ans. It should be dispensed in wide mouthed bottle because it is easy to take small amount of substance from a wide mouthed bottle.

Q. 16 Write the label for Mandl's paint.

FOR EXTERNAL USE ONLY

THE PAINT

Name   : Dinesh

Age   : 30

Sex   : Male

Regd. No. : 2130

Direction: Apply on throat with cotton swab, twice daily in between meals.

UCMS Pharmacy   *Anuj*
26/4/04

SHAKE WELL BEFORE USE

Q. 17 Write the prescription for Mandl's paint.

Dr. Rohit Arora
85, GTB Enclave
Regd. 2003/UCMS/007
Dated: 28-04-04

Begam Ali
35/Female
Regd. No. 3110

Δ   Pharyngitis

℞

I_2	-	250 mg
K1	-	500 mg
Water	-	0.5 ml
Oil of peppermint	-	0.08 ml
Alcohol	-	0.75 ml
Glycerine ad	-	20 ml

Mix well and send such 20 ml.

Apply in throat with cotton swab, twice daily, in between meals.

Rohit
Regd. 2003/UCMS/007

5. Carminative Mixture

Aim:

To prepare and dispense two doses of carminative mixture for an adult.

Apparatus:

Weighing balance with weights, glass mortar and pestle, measuring cylinder, dispensing bottle, cork, white paper cap, thread, wax paper, white paper, brown paper, chemicals.

Composition

Ingredients	For single adult dose
Sodium bicarbonate	0.6 gm
Spirit Ammonium aromaticus	1 ml
Tincture cardamom composita	1 ml
Tincture gingibaris	2 ml
Spirit chloroform	60 ml

Procedure:

Sodium bicarbonate was weighed on wax paper and ground in the mortar. The requisite amount of tincture cardamom co. and tincture gingibaris were added and mixed thoroughly. To this spirit ammonium aromaticus and spirit chloroform were added followed by sufficient amount of vehicle mixed and transferred to the dispensing bottle. The mortar and pestle were rinsed with more vehicle till the total volume becomes 60 ml. A cork, white paper cap and pharmaceutical knot were applied. Dose labels were put on one side. Labelling was done.

Viva Questions

Q. 1   What is a mixture?

Ans.   It is an aqueous preparation of medicament meant for oral use only.

Q. 2   What are the different types of mixture?

Ans.

(a) Simple: a clear solution without any precipitation even after prolonged standing e.g. carminative mixture.

(b) Diffusible: On standing, forms a suspension of solid particles eg. $Al(OH)_3$ gel.

(c) Non diffusible: Active ingredient is insoluble and does not form clear suspension even on shaking eg. Bismuth Kaolin mixture.

Q. 3   What are carminatives?

Ans.   These are drugs which promote expulsion of gases from the stomach by relaxing the lower esophageal sphincter (LES). They also give a feeling of warmth and relief in the abdomen by bringing about eructation.

      Examples: 1.   Sodium bicarbonate
                         2.   Oil of Peppermint
                         3.   Tincture cardamom
                         4.   Methyl polysiloxane.

Q. 4   What is the composition of carminative mixture?

Ans.

$NaHCO_3$	0.6 gm
Spirit ammonium aromaticus	1 ml
Tincture cardamom composita	1 ml
Tincture gingibaris	2 ml
Spirit chloroform	0.6 ml
Aqua ad	30 ml

This is the composition of 1 dose.

Q. 5   What are the carminative principles in this preparation.

Ans. $NaHCO_3$, Spirit ammonium aromatics, Tincture cardamon composita.

Q. 6   What is tincture cardamom composed of?
1. Cinnamon (Dalchini)
2. Cardamom (Elaichi)
3. Caraway
4. Glycerine
5. Alcohol
6. Extract of cochineal insect (imparts red colour)

Q. 7   What is the composition of spirit ammonium aromaticus?

Ans. NH_4HCO_3, strong solution of NH_3, Oil of lemon, alcohol, oil of nutmeg and water.

Q. 8   How does $NaHCO_3$ act as a carminative?

Ans. $NaHCO_3$ reacts with HCl in stomach to produce CO_2.

$$NAHCO_3 + HCl \Rightarrow NaCl + H_2O + CO_2$$

This CO_2 is responsible for relaxing the LES.

Q. 9   Describe the individual functions of each ingredient.

Ans.

(a) $NaHCO_3$-Releases CO_2. Thereby relaxing the LES and distending the stomach thus causing eructation.

(b) Spirit ammonium aromatics: Relaxes LES.

(c) Tincture cardamom composita: Irritates gastric mucosa thus increasing gastrointestinal motility, also relaxes the LES

(d) Tincture gingibaris: Relaxes LES

(e) Spirit chloroform: Increases shelf life, provides flavour.

Q. 10 Name the uses of carminative mixture.

1. Flatulent dyspepsia

2. To prevent regurgitation of milk in infants.

Q. 11 Why is it given after meals?

Ans. There is more accumulation of gases after meals, so it is more effective after meals.

Q. 12 How is the dose label put?

Ans. A narrow strip of paper is cut, whose length is equal to the height of the mixture in the dispensing bottle.

The strip of paper is folded end to end and the corners of the folded end are nicked. The strip is then unfolded and pasted vertically on the centre of the dispensing bottle on the marked side. [Fig. I(1)]

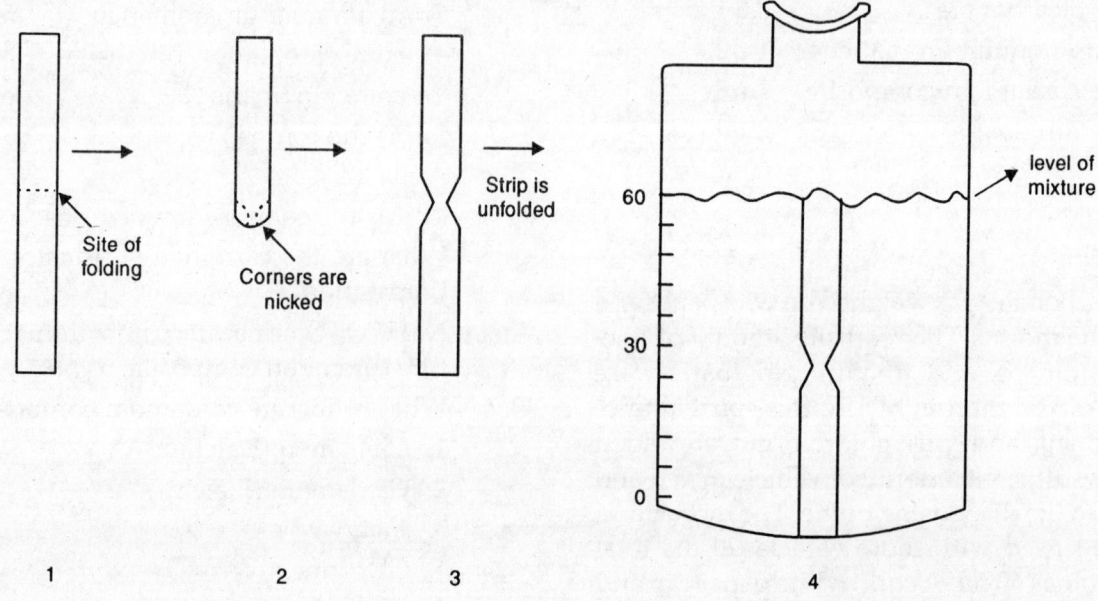

Fig. I(1)

Q. 13 Write the label for the preparation.

THE MIXTURE

Name   : Sumit Lal

Age   : 58

Sex   : Male

Regd. No. : 025

Directions: One dose to be taken twice daily after meals.

UCMS Pharmacy   *Roshan*
09.05.04

Q. 14. Write the prescription for carminative mixture

Dr. Arun Dutt
B-11/Sec 3, Rohini
Regd. No. 01/05/4443
Dated: 09-05-04

Mahipal Singh
50 yr/Male
Regd. No. 216

Δ Flatulent dyspepsia

℞

$NaHCO_3$	0.6 gm
Spirit ammonium aromaticus	1 ml
Tincture Cardamom composita	1 ml
Tincture Gingibaris	2 ml
Spirit Chloroform	0.6 ml
Aqua ad.	30 ml

Send such 60 ml.

One dose of 30 ml to be taken twice daily after meals.

Arun
Regd. No. 01/05/4443

6. Tincture Iodine

Aim:

To prepare and dispense 20 ml of tincture iodine.

Apparatus:

Weighing balance with weights, glass mortar and pestle, measuring cylinder, blue dispensing bottle with glass stopper, red cap, thread, white paper, wax paper, brown paper, chemicals.

Composition:

Ingredients for 20 ml

Iodine	400 mg
Potassium iodide	500 mg
Alcohol (50%) ad	20 ml

Procedure:

The requisite amount of iodine was weighed, ground in glass mortar. Then potassium iodide was weighed and ground. To this a small amount of alcohol was added to make a solution. The solution was then transferred to a measuring cylinder. The mortar and pestle were rinsed with sufficient amount of alcohol to make the total volume upto 20 ml. A red paper cap and pharmaceutical knot was put. Labelling was done as follows.

Viva Questions

Q. 1 What is a tincture.

Ans. These are alcoholic or hydroalcoholic solutions of the active principles obtained from vegetable or chemical sources. Most of the tinctures are obtained from maceration, percolation or dilution of a more concentrated preparations.

Q. 2 Name the tinctures made for external use.

Ans. 1. Tincture iodine
2. Tincture Benzoin

Q. 3 Name the tincture for internal use.

Ans. 1. Tincture cardamom composita
2. Tincture Belladona
3. Tincture digitalis

Q. 4 What is the difference between Spirits and Liquors.

Ans. Spiritis are alcoholic or hydroalcoholic solutions of the volatile substances eg. spirit ammonium aromaticus, spirit chloroform.

Liquors are solutions of non-volatile medicinal substances in water or alcohol eg. liquor morphine, liquor iodi mitis (Tincture iodine).

Q. 5 What is the other name of Tincture Iodine?

Ans. Liquor iodi mitis.

Q. 6 What is the composition of Tincture Iodine?

Ans.

	100 ml	20 ml
Iodine	2g	400 mg
Pottasium Iodide	2.5 g	500 mg
Alcohol (50%) ad.	100 ml	20 ml

Q. 7 What are the uses of the ingredients?

Ans. *Iodine*: It acts as antiseptic and bactericidal. It reacts with pottasium iodide to liberate nascent iodine which is responsible for oxidation.

$$I_2 + KI \longrightarrow KI_3 \longrightarrow KII + 2[I]$$

Pottasium Iodide - Used to dissolve iodine.

Alcohol: (a) Stabilizes the solution.
(b) acts as a vehicle.
(c) aids quick drying.
(d) mild antiseptic
(e) preservative.

Q. 8 What are other preparations of iodine.

Ans. (a) Mandl's Paint
(b) Liquid iodi fortis
(c) Lugol's iodine
(d) Non straining iodine ointment
(e) Radioactive iodine

Q. 9   Write the label for Tincture Iodine.

Ans.

FOR EXTERNAL USE ONLY

<u>THE TINCTURE</u>

Name   : Sunil

Age   : 24 yrs.

Sex   : Male

Regd. No. : 1362

Directions: To be applied on affected part, when required.

UCMS Pharmacy   *Rajesh*
12.07.2004

10. Write the prescription of Tincture iodine.

Ans.

Dr. Sunil Gautam
30 A, Pocket-A
Delhi-110093
Regd. No. 16/2004/732
Dated: 12.07.2004

Sunil
24/Male
Regd. No. 1362

Δ Abrasion

℞

Iodine	2g
Pottasium iodide	2.5 g
Alcohol ad.	100 ml

Mix and make and send such 20 ml. Apply on the affected part, when required.

Sunil
Regd. No. 16/2004/732

---

7. Liniment Turpentine

Aim:

To prepare and disperse 25 ml of turpentine liniment.

Apparatus:

Weighing balance with weights, porcelain mortar and pestle, measuring cylinder, blue bottle, paper cap, wax paper, brown and white papers, chemicals.

Composition	
Ingredients	For 25 ml
Turpentine oil	16.5 ml
Soft soap	1.87 gm
Camphor	1.25 gm
Aqua ad	25 ml

Procedure:

The requisite amount of camphor was weighed, finely powdered, and mixed with soft soap in a mortar. Oil of turpentine was added to it gradually, triturating well after each addition. The mixture was then transferred to a blue bottle with the aid of distilled water and shaken thoroughly after each addition until a creamy emulsion was formed. Red paper cap and pharmaceutical knot was applied. Labelling of the bottle was done as follows.

Viva Questions

Q. 1   What is a liniment?

Ans.   It is an aquous or oily preparation of medicament which is applied on affected part by rubbing.

Q. 2   What is the difference between ointment and liniment?

Ans.   Both are meant for external use but liniment is applied on the affected part by rubbing whereas ointment need not be rubbed.

Q. 3   What is the composition of liniment Turpentine.

Ans.   For 25 ml

Turpentine Oil	16.5 ml
Soft Soap	1.87 g
Camphor	1.25 g
Aqua ad.	25 ml

Q. 4   What are the uses of ingredients?

Ans.   Turpentine oil – acts as a counter-irritant.
Soft Soap – as emulsifying agent.
Camphor – vasodilation.

Q. 5   What is meant by counter irritant?

Ans.   These are irritants which when applied locally on skin helps in relieving the deep seated pain.

Q. 6   How do counter-irritant act?

Ans.   These act by two mechanisms.

(1)   On application to the skin, these stimulates the sensory nerve endings in the skin and this impulse interferes with the transmission of pain impulse coming from deep structures within the same segmented level. Thus counter irritants results in partial or complete exclusion of pain impulse from deep structures by occupying the final common pathway.

(2)   Also vasodilation occurs in the deep structures supplied by same segmented level as the skin, where counter-irritants are applied. Hence, metabolites responsible for pain such as substance P are removed due to increased blood flow.

Q. 7   What are various types of irritants?

Ans.   Irritants are substances which produce changes in cellular structures and are capable of producing inflammation. According to degree of inflammation produced, these are classified as
Rubifacient – produce redness.
Vesicants   – produce vesicles.
Pustulants – pustules are produced.

Q. 8   Why liniment is applied by rubbing?

Ans.   By rubbing, heat is produced which results in vasodilation and thus more of the metabolites are removed due to increased blood flow.

Q. 9   What are the uses of this preparation?

Ans.   It is used to relieve deep seated pain like arthralgia (joint pain), myaglia (muscular pain), neuralgia (nerve pain) etc.

Q. 10 Why it should not be applied on broken skin?

Ans.   Because if applied on broken skin, it gets absorbed and acts as irritant to deep structures also.

Q. 11 Write the label for this preparation.

FOR EXTERNAL USE ONLY

THE LINIMENT

Name – Sunder

Age – 26 years

Sex – Male

Regd. No. – 1624

Directions: Apply on the affected area by rubbing

UCMS Pharmacy   *Ramesh*
12:07:2004

SHOULD NOT BE APPLIED ON BROKEN SKIN

Q. 12. Write the prescription of Turpentine liniment.

Ans.

Dr. Rakesh Mittal
27, Block-B, Rohini
Delhi-110067
Regd. No. 62/2004/72
Dated: 12/07/2004

Name   : Sunder
Age/Sex   : 26 yr/Male
Regd. No. : 1624

Δ - Myalgia

R

Turpentine Oil	16.5 ml
Soft Soap	1.87 g
Camphor	1.25 g
Aqua ad.	25 ml

Mix and make and send such 25 ml.

Apply on the affected area by rubbing.

Rakesh
Regd. No. 62/2004/72

8. Whitfield Ointment

Aim:

To prepare and dispense 25 gm of whitfield ointment.

Apparatus:

Same as in case of sulphur ointment.

Composition:

Ingredients	For 25 gm
Benzoic acid	1.5 gm
Salicylic acid	0.75 gm
Simple ointment	22.75 gm

Procedure:

Same as in case of sulphur ointment. Labelling is done as follows.

Q. 1 What is an ointment?

Ans. It is semi solid greasy preparation of medicament which is meant for external use only.

Q. 2 What is the composition of this preparation?

Ans. For 25 g

Benzoic Acid	1.5 g
Salicylic Acid	0.75 g
Simple Ointment	22.75 g

Q. 3 What are the uses of ingredients?

Ans. Benzoic Acid – Antifungal

Salicylic Acid – Keratolytic and antifungal

Simple Ointment – It is composed of

Hard Paraffin – provide consistency to ointment

Wool Fat – Hydrophilic so increases absorption of medicament

Soft Paraffin – Emulsifying agent.

Q. 4 What is the use of Whitfield Ointment?

Ans. It is used for treatment of superficial fungal infections like dermatophytosis e.g. tinea pedis, tinea corporis, tinea cruris, tinea versicolor etc.

Q. 5 What is the use of keratolytic agent?

Ans. Keratolytic agents like salicylic acid causes the lysis of keratin and thus helps in the better absorption of the drug.

Q. 6 Name other antifungal drugs.

Ans. 1. *Antibiotics*: Amphotericin B, Nystatin, Greisofulvin.

2. *Azoles*:

(a) Imidazoles: Clotrimazole, Econazole, Miconazole, Ketoconazole.

(b) Triazoles: Fluconazole, Intraconazole

3. *Antimetabolites*: Flucytosine

4. *Alkylamine*: Terbinafine

5. *Miscellaneous*: Tolnaftate, Whitfield Ointment.

Q. 7 What are the main side effects of Amphotericin B?

Ans. a. Nephrotoxicity

b. Acute Reaction on iv. administration due to release of histamine

c. Anemia

Q. 8 What are newer preparations of Amphoterin B?

Ans. (a) Amphotericin B Lipid Complex (ABCL)

(b) Amphotericin B Colloidal Dispersion (ABCD)

(c) Liposomal Amphotericin B.

Q. 9 Why these newer preparations are formed?

Ans. These are formed to counteract the side-effects of Amphotericin B. These preparations result in better tolerability by decreasing the acute reaction on i/v infusion.

• Lesser Nephortoxicity

• Lesser Anemia

Q. 10 Name some other ointment.

Ans. Sulphur ointment used for scabies.

Q. 11 In which container, Whitfield ointment is dispensed?

Ans. Pill Box.

Q. 12 Write the Label for this preparation.

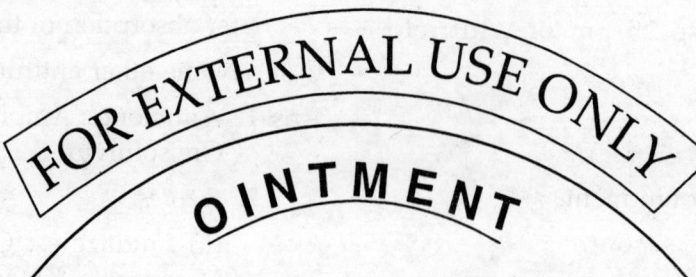

FOR EXTERNAL USE ONLY

OINTMENT

Name   : Sanjay
Age   : 24 yrs.
Sex   : Male
Regd. No. : 1712

Direction: To be applied on affected
                    part twice daily.

UCMS Pharmacy   *Sanjay*
12.07.2004

Q. 13 Write the prescription of Whitfield Ointment.

Ans.

Dr. Sanjeev Mann
16/32, Dilshad Colony
Delhi-110095.
Regd. No. 612/2004/763
Dated: 12-07-04

Sanjay
24 yr/M
Regd. No. 1634

Δ - Tinea corporis

℞

Benzoic Acid	1.5 g
Salicylic Acid	0.75 g
Simple Ointment	22.75 g

Mix and make and send such 25 g.

Apply on the affected part twice daily.

Sanjeev
Regd. No. 612/2004/763

9. Benzyl Benzoate Emulsion

Aim:

To prepare and dispense 23 ml of Benzylbenzoate emulsion.

Apparatus:

Weighing balance with weights, porcelain mortal and pestle, measuring cylinder, dispensing bottle with cork, paper cap, wax paper, brown and white paper, chemicals.

Composition:

Ingredients for 25 ml

Benzyl benzoate	6.25 ml
Emulsifying wax	500 mg
Aqua ad	25 ml

Procedure:

The emulsifying wax was heated in a china dish and 6.25 ml benzyl benzoate was added. The liquid was transferred to a measuring cylinder and hot water was added till the final volume was 25 ml. Finally the preparation was transferred to a wide mouthed bottle and shaken vigorously.

Viva Questions

Q. 1   What is an emulsion?

Ans.   It is a mixture of two immiscible liquids in which one is finely divided and uniformly distributed throughout the other liquid with the help of an emulsifying agent.

Q. 2   What is dispersed phase and continuous phase?

Ans.   The liquid which is finely divided and is less in amount is in dispersed phase whereas the liquid in large amount in which the dispersed phase is present, is in continuous phase.

Q. 3   What is function of emulsifying agent?

Ans.   It forms the coating around each particle and prevents coalescence with one another.

Q. 4   What are various types of emulsifying agents?

Ans.   a. Gums eg. gum acacia

b. Protein eg. egg yolk, caesin of milk

c. Soaps

d. emulsifying wax, wool fat

e. agar-agar

Q. 5   Describe various types of emulsions with examples.

Ans.   There are two types of emulsions.

1. Oil in water

2. Water in oil.

(1) **Oil in water**: In this type of emulsion, oil is in less quantity and is dispersed in the water, which acts as continuous phase eg. benzyl benzoate emulsion, milk, castor oil emulsion, shark liver oil emulsion.

(2) **Water in Oil:** In this type of emulsion, water is in small quantity and is dispersed in oil, which acts as continuous phase, e.g. cold cream, hair cream etc.

Q. 6   What is meant by cracking of emulsion?

Ans.   When the substance in dispersed phase is not properly dispersed or does not remain dispersed, it is known as cracking of emulsion.

Q. 7   What can be the causes of cracking?

Ans.   (a) Excessive Heating or Cooling.

(b) pH changes

(c) growth of bacteria

Q. 8   What is meant by creaming of emulsion?

Ans.   When the two layers of the liquid separate out according to their densities, it is known as creaming of emulsion. However, on shaking the bottle, emulsion becomes continuous.

Q. 9   What is the cause of creaming of emulsion?

Ans.   It is due to improper method of making of emulsion.

Q. 10 What precaution do you take while preparing emulsion?

Ans.   While mixing the liquids, the stirring should be done only in one direction.

Q. 11 Why are emulsions white in colour?

Ans.   Because of Tyndal's effect, all the light rays are reflected by the emulsion, and thus the reflected light falling on the eyes has light of all wavelengths, so appears white.

Q. 12 What are the advantages of making emulsions?

Ans.

(a) To make the drug more palatable by masking its taste and smell.

(b) Insoluble drugs are made soluble by emulsifying agent.

(c) By increasing the surface area (due to presence of the medicament in finely divided state), absorption of the drug is enhanced.

Q. 13 Which type of emulsion have you prepared in this experiment?

Ans. Oil in water.

Q. 14 How do you test the type of emulsion?

Ans. *Water in Oil Type*: On adding oil (continuous phase) to the emulsion, it becomes diluted and on adding water (dispersed phase), it get cracked.

Oil in Water type: On adding water (continuous phase), to the emulsion, it only becomes diluted whereas on adding oil, it cracks.

In brief, add water to the emulsion to be tested, if it becomes diluted it is oil in water emulsion whereas if it get cracked, it is water in oil emulsion.

Q. 15 What is the use of Benzyl benzoate emulsion?

Ans. It is used for treatment of scabies.

Q. 16 Which organism causes scabies?

Ans. It is caused by a mite, sarcoptes scabei.

Q. 17 How is benzyl benzoate emulsion applied?

Ans. It should be applied all over the body except face and neck, after a hot scrubbed bath. It is reapplied next day and washed after 24 hours.

Q. 18 What are the main precautions taken for the treatment of scabies?

Ans. 1. Benzyl benzoate emulsion should be applied after hot scrubbed bath.

2. All members of the family and other persons who are in close contact with the patient should also be treated simultaneously.

3. The clothings and beddings etc. are washed in boiling water.

Q. 19 Why the hot scrubbed bath is necessary before application of benzyl benzoate?

Ans. Because, after hot scrubbed bath, the burrows of the mite are opened and the drug can reach the mite easily.

Q. 20 Why all contacts of the patient are treated simultaneously?

Ans. Because, it is a very contagious disease and if any person in contact is left untreated, it will again attack all the members.

Q. 21 Name other drugs used for the treatment of scabies?

Ans. Permethrin (5%)

• Lindane (γ-Benzene hexachloride or gammaxene) - 1%

• Benzyl benzoate emulsion - 25%

• Crotamiton - 10%

• Sulphur Ointment.

Q. 22 Which part of body scabies affect the most?

Ans. Scabies is seen mostly in fexural areas like interdigital clefts, elbow joints, armpits etc.

Q. 23 Write the label for Benzyl benzoate emulsion.
Ans.

FOR EXTERNAL USE ONLY

<u>THE EMULSION</u>

Name   : Bittoo
Age   : 1½ yr
Sex   : M
Regd. No. : 1862

Directions: Apply all over the body below neck after a hot scrubbed bath, repeat application after 12 hours followed by a bath with the change of clothings.

UCMS Pharmacy   *Rajeev*
12.07.2004

SHAKE WELL BEFORE USE

Q. 24 Write the prescription of Benzyl benzoate emulsion.

Ans.

Dr. Sulabh Goel
6/27, Shastri Nagar
Delhi-110067
Regd. No.-121/2004/361

Bittoo
1½ yr/M
Regd. No. 1862

Δ - Scabies

℞

Benzyl benzoate	6.25 ml
Emulsifying wax	500 mg
Aqua ad.	25 ml

Mix and make and send such 25 ml.

Apply all over the body below neck after hot scrubbed bath, repeat application after 12 hours followed by a bath with change of clothings.

12.07.2004   *Sulabh*
                                   Regd. No.-121/2004/361

10. Oral Rehydration Salt

Aim:

To prepare and dispense oral rehydration salt for 1000 ml solution.

Apparatus:

Balance with fractional weights, tile, spatula, wax paper, scissors, ruler and chemicals.

Composition:

It is a mixture of following ingredients.

Sodium chloride	3.5 g
Potassium chloride	1.5 g
Trisodium citrate	2.9 g
Glucose	20 g
Water	1000 ml

Procedure:

The above ingredients are measured and taken on the tile. Mixing is done using spatula. An inner packing of white paper measuring 3"× 5" and an outer packing of brown paper measuring 5"× 7" is done. Labelling is then done on the outer packet.

Viva Questions

Q. 1 What is a powder?

Ans. It is a medicament which is finely ground and wrapped in a paper so that each wrapping represents one dose of a drug.

Q. 2 What are various types of powders?

Ans. *Simple Powder:* In this, one medicament is powdered and dispensed e.g. aspirin.

Compound Powder: Two or more medicaments are dispensed together in same wrapping because combination has to be given e.g. In APC powder, acetylsalicylic acid, paracetamol and caffeine are dispensed together.

Fractional Powder: In this, medicament is in very low doses (in fractions of mg) e.g. Hyoscine hydrobromide powder.

Q. 3 What is the composition of ORS?

Ans.
Sodium chloride	– 3.5g
Potassium chloride	– 1.5g
Trisodium citrate	– 2.9g
Glucose	– 20g
Water	– 1000 ml

Q. 4 What is the concentration of constituents in mmols?

Ans.
Na^+	– 90 mM
K^+	– 20 mM
Cl^-	– 80 mM
Citrate	– 10 mM
Glucose	– 111 mM
Osmolality	– 311 mOsm/L

Q. 5 In which condition it is used?

Ans. It is used for mild or moderate diarrhoea.

Q. 6 Why is it not given in severe diarrhoea?

Ans. Because in severe diarrhoea, there is severe dehydration and so quick improvement of hydration is required which is not possible with oral solution. Thus in severe diarrhoea, intravenous fluids are given first.

Q. 7 The composition of ORS prepared by you is based on which diarrhoea?

Ans. It is based on the composition of stool of "diarrohea due to cholera".

Q. 8 What is "New Formula WHO-ORS"?

Ans. WHO released Low Na^+ low glucose formula in 2002. It is based on stool composition of Enterotoxigenic E.coli (ETEC) diarrhoea.

Its composition is

Na^+	– 75 mM
K^+	– 20 mM
Cl^-	– 65 mM
Citrate	– 10 mM
Glucose	– 75 mM
Osmolality	– 245 mM

NaCl	– 2.6 g
KCl	– 1.5 g
Trisodium citrate	– 2.9 g
Glucose	– 13.5 g
Water	– 1000 ml

Q. 9 What is the reason for this modification in WHO ORS?

Ans. 1. Na^+ has been decreased from 90 mM to 75 mM because it has been seen that in some patients, WHO-ORS produced periorbital edema due to excess Na^+.

2. Glucose has been reduced from 110 mM to 75 mM because in some patients WHO-ORS produced increase in stool volume due to osmotic activity of glucose in colon.

3. WHO-ORS was based on stool composition of cholera stools in children. But as the cases of cholera has been decreased considerably, these drawbacks are seen.

Q. 10 What are the non-diarrhoeal uses of ORS?

Ans. 1. Maintenance of hydration and nutrition after surgery, burn or trauma.

2. Heat stroke

3. During changeover from Total Parenteral Nutrition to enteral nutrition.

Q. 11 What are the functions of ingredients?

Ans. Glucose – helps in absorption of Na^+ because of intactness of Glucose mediated Na^+ absorption.

$\left.\begin{matrix} Na^+ \\ K^+ \end{matrix}\right]$ –For maintaining electrolyte and fluid balance.

Citrate – For combating acidosis.

Q. 12 What is Super ORS?

Ans. This is a solution which, in addition to maintaining hydration also decreases diarrhoea, by enhancing absorption. It can be made by

(a) adding certain amino acids like alanine, glycine etc.

(b) By replacing glucose with boiled rice powder.

Q. 13 Why was sodium bicarbonate replaced by sodium citrate in ORS?

Ans. Because sodium bicarbonate reacts with glucose to form furfural compounds which imparts brown colours to the salt.

Q. 14 What are the general principles followed during formulation of ORS?

Ans. 1. It should be isotonic or somewhat hypotonic to plasma (i.e. osmolality in 210-300 mosm/L) because diarrhoeal fluids are approximately isotonic with plasma.

2. Glucose should be equal or somewhat higher than Na^+ because excess glucose will help in absorbing Na^+ present in intestinal secretions in addition to that present in ORS.

3. K^+ and base (citrate/bicarbonate) should be enough to covers the losses in stool.

Q. 15 How in ORS administered?

Ans. One packet of ORS is mixed in half litre of water and patient in instructed to drink as much as he can after every stool.

Q. 16 How is ORS dispensed.

Ans. It is dispensed in a packet. The required composition is first put in an inner pack which is then covered by an outer pack.

Q. 17 Write the label for ORS.

THE POWDER

Name   :   Sonu

Age   :   7 yr.

Sex   :   Male

Regd. No. :   A 212

Directions – One pack is dissolved in half litre of water and should be taken after every stool.

UCMS Pharmacy   *Vinod*
12.07.2004

Q. 18 Write the prescription of ORS.

Ans.

Dr. Tarun Arora
12/26, Shastri Nagar
Delhi-110062
Regd. No. 112/UCMS/05
Dated: 12.05.2004

Sonu
2 yr/M
Regd. No. 12/4

Δ - Diarrhoea

℞

Sodium Chloride	1.75 mg
Pottasium Chloride	0.75 mg
Trisodium Citrate	1.45 mg
Glucose	10 mg

Mix and send 2 such packets.

Dissolve 1 packet in 500 ml of water and drink as much as possible after every stool.

Tarun
Regd. No. 112/UCMS/05

11. Hyoscine Hydrobromide Powder

Aim:

To prepare and dispense 4 doses of hyoscine hydrobromide powder each containing 0.3 mg of HHBr.

Apparatus:

Balance with fractional weights, tile, spatula, wax paper, scissors, ruler and chemicals.

Procedure:

Mixing of the ingredients was done in ascending order as follows:-

1. 100 mg of HHBr was mixed with 900 mg of lactose = Powder A
2. 100 mg of A was mixed with 900 mg of lactose = Powder B
3. 150 mg of powder B was mixed with 850 mg of lactose = Powder C.
4. 4 packets of Powder C made each one containing 200 mg.

   Packing of the 4 inner packets is done as follows:

   Four pieces of wax paper was cut each measuring 3" × 5". It was folded in 2 parts so that one part is slightly bigger than the other (length wise), the powder being kept at the centre. The extra bit of paper was now folded over the short paper and the whole paper was then folded into two unequal halves. The two ends were then folded inwards so that they lie in apposition and the side with the unequal fold outside.

   The outer packet is made as follows:

   A piece of white paper was cut measuring 5" × 7". The 4 packets were kept on the paper in such a way that they are facing upwards. The paper was now folded in the same way except for the last fold; while folding the two ends, one should be made longer than the other and the shorter one was pushed inside the longer fold and the labelling was done.

Viva Questions

Q. 1   What type of powder is HHBr?

Ans.   It is a fractional powder.

Q. 2   What is the use of HHBr Powder?

Ans.   1. To prevent motion sickness.

Q. 3   How does HHBr prevent motion sickness? It acts by

1. Depressing CNS
2. Inhibits the initiation of impulses from semi-circular canals and over stimulation of vestibular apparatus and medulla. It suppresses excessive vagal activity. It is useful only for prophylactic treatment.

Q. 4.   What are the side effects of HHBr powder?

Ans.   1. Dryness of mouth
2. Dilation of pupil thus causing blurring of vision.
3. Difficulty in micturition
4. Sedation
5. Amnesia

Q. 5.   What other drugs are used in motion sickness.

Ans.

i) Antihistaminics :	Promethazine
	Cyclizine
	Meclizine
ii) Anti-dopaminergics:	Chlorpromazine
	Prochlorperazine
	Metochlorpramide
iii) Miscellaneous	Pyridoxine
	Amphetamines

Q. 6.   Why is the powder made in the given manner i.e. A, B, C?

Ans.   Because the amount of HHBr is very less. So this is the only way to dilute it.

Q. 7.   Write the label for this preparation.

THE POWDER

Name   : Sudesh

Age   : 20 yrs.

Regd. No.   : 3126

Directions: Take one dose half an hour before journey, and repeat a dose after 4 hours if needed.

UCMS Pharmacy   *Ramesh*
7.5.04

Q. 8.   Write the prescription?

Ans.

Dr. Mohit
B-6/151 Sec-11 Rohini
Regd. No. 04/562
Dated: 12-10-03

Nalini
18 yr/Female
Regd. No. 2112

Δ - Motion sickness

℞

Hyoscine hydrobromide powder - 0.3 mg

Send such 4 packets.

Take one dose (packet) half an hour before journey and repeat after 4 hours if needed.

Mohit
Regd. No. 04/562

12. APC Powder

Aim:

To prepare and dispense 3 doses of APC Powder.

Apparatus:

Balance with fractional weights, tile, spatula, white paper, envelope.

Composition:

APC powder is a mixture of the following drugs.

Ingredients	1 Dose	3 Doses	4 Doses
1. Acetyl Salicylic acid	200 mg	600 mg	800 mg
2. Phenacetin	150 mg	450 mg	600 mg
3. Caffeine citrate	30 mg	90 mg	120 mg

Procedure:

The above ingredients are mixed in an ascending order i.e. caffeine first followed by phenacetin and then aspirin, each being weighed and mixed in the following way:

120 mg of caffeine + 120 mg of Phenacetin = A

A + 240 mg Phenacetin = B

B + 240 mg Phenacetin + 240 mg Aspirin = C

C + 560 mg Aspirin = D.

Now 3 doses of 'D' powder each weighing 380 mg were made. The rest was discarded. An inner packing of white paper measuring 3″ × 5″ and an outer packing of brown paper measuring 5″ × 7″ is done. Labelling is then done on the outer packet as follows.

THE POWDER

Name   : Shanti

Age   : 30 yrs

Regd No.: 4126

Directions: One dose to be taken after meal.

UCMS Pharmacy   *Monty*
3.5.98

Viva Questions

Q. 1 What are the uses of the constituents of APC powder?

1. Acetyl salicylic acid (Aspirin) – It is an analgesic, antipyretic, as well as anti-inflammatory agent.
2. Phenacetin – It is also analgesic and antipyretic.
3. Caffeine – It is a CNS stimulant used to elevate the mood of the patient. It also causes constriction of the cerebral blood vessels thereby getting rid of headache.

Q. 2 What are the indications of APC powder?

1. Fever
2. Headache
3. Dull aching superficial pains like neuralgia, myalgia, arthralgia and toothache. It is not useful in deep seated visceral and shooting pains.

Q. 3 What is the dose of aspirin for analgesia?

Ans. 0.3-1 gm

Q. 4 Why is APC powder given after meals?

Ans. Because it irritates the gastric mucosa, causing excessive HCl production and may cause gastric ulcer. Hence it is always given after food.

Q. 5 Why is the dose of phenacetin less than aspirin inspite of being equipotent?

Ans. Because phenacitin has an additive effect when given in combination with aspirin.

Q. 6 What is the mechanism of action of aspirin?

Ans. Aspirin inhibits the enzyme cyclooxygenase thereby blocking the synthesis of prostaglandins. Decreased production of prostaglandins resets the thermostat of the body (present in the hypothalamus) thereby lowering the temperature.

Q. 7 Write the prescription for APC Powder.

Dr. Arshad,
74, Vasant Kunj,
Regd. No. 4125/UCMS/25
Dated: 8-5-2004

Sudhir Kumar
18 yr/Male
Regd. No. 3166

Δ - Pyrexia of unknown origin

℞

Acetyl salicylic acid	600 mg
Phenacetin	450 mg
Caffeine citrate	90 mg

Mix the above and divide into 3 doses.
Take one dose after every meal.

Arshad
Regd. No. 4.25/UCMS/25

13. Castor Oil Emulsion

Aim:

To prepare and dispense two doses of castor oil emulsion for a child of 10 years.

Apparatus:

Weighing balance with weights, porcelain mortar and pestle, measuring cylinder, dispensing bottle with cork, paper cap, wax paper, brown and white paper chemicals.

Composition:

Ingredients required for 10 ml of oil are:

Castor oil	10 ml
Water	5 ml
Gum acacia	2.5 gm

Procedure:

There are two different methods of preparing castor oil emulsion, dry gum and wet gum methods. For both the methods the proportions of ingredients are the same i.e.

Fixed oil (i.e. castor oil)	:	4 parts
Water	:	2 parts
Gum	:	1 part

(a) Wet gum method: The required amount of powdered gum is taken into the mortar and water is added gradually. Then oil is added until all the oil has been incorporated. Finally the volume is made up by adding other ingredients and the vehicle.

(b) Dry gum method: The gum is first mixed with oil after which the volume is made by adding other ingredients and the vehicle.

The emulsion is dispensed in a dispensing bottle and a white cap is tied with a pharmaceutical knot, labelling of the bottle is done as follows.

THE EMULSION

Name   : Sunil
Age   : 10 yrs.
Regd. No. : 7124

Directions: One dose to be taken early in the morning on empty stomach.

UCMS Pharmacy
8-8-2004   *Manish*

SHAKE WELL BEFORE USE

Viva Questions

Q. 1 What are the indications of castor oil emulsion?

Ans. It is an irritant purgative given orally in cases of constipation.

Q. 2 What is the mechanism of action of castor oil?

Ans. It is a triglyceride of ricinoleic acid, obtained from castor seed (Ricinus communis). It is an emolient when applied locally on skin, but an irritant purgative when given orally. Castor oil is broken down by pancreatic lipase into glycerol and ricinoleic acid. This combines with alkali of the intestinal juice and forms alkali ricinoleate, which increases intestinal motility and causes evacuation of bowel. Onset of action is 1-3 hours and duration is 6 hours.

Q. 3 Why is castor oil given in the morning?

Ans. Because the onset of action of castor oil is 6 hours.

Q. 4 What kind of emulsion is castor oil?

Ans. Castor oil is an "oil in water" type of emulsion. In this type of emulsion, the oil is less in amount and is present in a dispersed form while water is present in a continuous phase.

Q. 5 What are the other examples of oil in water emulsions?

Ans. Milk, shark liver oil, and benzyl benzoate.

Q. 6 Why is a white cap used?

Ans. Because castor oil emulsion is not for external use. It is for internal use.

Q. 7 What precautions should be taken while making this emulsion?

Ans. 1. Dry and separate measuring glasses should be used for oil and water.

2. Porcelain mortar and pestles are used.

3. Emulsion is to be mixed in one direction only.

4. The oil should be added very slowly to the emulsion or it will crack.

5. A white paper cap is used.

Q. 8 Write a prescription for castor oil emulsion.

Dr. K.P. Singh
5/Vasant Vihar
Regd. No. 05/UCMS/95
Dated: 8-05-04

Suhail Ali
27/M
Regd. No. 420.

Δ - Constipation

Castor oil	10 ml
Water	5 ml
Gum acacia	2.5 gm

Mix and send such 10 ml.
One dose to be taken early morning on empty stomach.

Kailash
Regd. No. 05/UCMS/95

---

14. Shark Liver Oil Emulsion

Aim:

To prepare and dispense 50 ml of shark liver oil emulsion.

Apparatus:

Weighing balance with weights, porcelain mortar and pestle, measuring cylinder, dispensing bottle with cork, paper cap, wax paper, brown and white paper, chemicals.

Composition:

Ingredients	For 100 ml	For 50 ml
Shark liver oil	25 ml	12.5 ml
Tragacanth, in powder	0.5 gm	0.25 gm
Acacia	6.25 gm	3.12 gm
Water up to	100 ml	50 ml

Procedure:

The emulsion is prepared by wet gum method, as described in the previous experiment. Labelling of the bottle is done as follows.

THE EMULSION

Name   : Tarun Arora

Age   : 26 yrs.

Regd. No. : 9015

Directions: One teaspoonful to be taken three times a day.

UCMS Pharmacy   *Rohit*
16.5.04

SHAKE WELL BEFORE USE

Viva Questions

Q. 1. What type of emulsion is shark liver oil?

Ans. It is an oil in water type of emulsion.

Q. 2. What are the indications of shark liver oil?

Ans. It contains vitamin A so it can be used in prophylaxis is of vitamin A deficiency disorders.

Q. 3. What is the amount of Vit A present is shark liver oil?

Ans. 6000 units in 1 gm.

Q. 4. What are thee symptoms of Vit A deficiency?
1. Night blindness
2. Bitot's spots
3. Xeropthalmia
4. Keratomalacia
5. Follicular hyperkeratosis

Q. 5. What are the symptoms of hyper vitaminosis A.

Ans. Irritability, loss of appetite, itching and hyper prothroinbinaemia.

Q. 6. What precautions are to be taken while making this emulsion.

Ans. Same as in previous experiment.

Q. 7. What is the function of tragacanth?

Ans. It is a stabilizer.

Q. 8. Write the prescription for shark liver oil.

Ans.

Dr. Munish Singh
15, Dilshad Garden
Reg. No. 00/UCMS/95
Dated: 9-05-04

Raghubir
04/Male
Reg No. 444

Δ - Night blindness

Shark Liver oil	12.5ml
Tragacanth	0.25gm
Acacia	6.25gm
Water ad.	50ml

Mix the above and send 50ml.

One teaspoonful to be taken thrice daily.

Munish
Regd No. 00/UCMS/99

15. Sulphur Ointment

Aim:

To prepare and dispense 20 gm of sulphur ointment(10%)

Apparatus:

Weighing balance with weights, china dish, water bath, porcelain tile, spatula, pill box, wax paper, white paper, chemicals.

Composition:

10% Sulphur ointment contains

Sublimed sulphur	2gm
Simple ointment	18 gm

Simple ointment contents

1. Hard paraffin	1.35 gm
2. Wool fat	1.35 gm
3. Yellow soft paraffin	15.30 gm

Procedure:

The required amount of sublimed sulphur was taken on one side of the porcelain tile and the simple ointment was poured on the other side; and the sulphur was thoroughly stirred with a spatula, till it was smooth. It was then dispensed in a pill box, the upper surface was made smooth and covered with wax paper. Lid was kept on it. The extra wax paper was cut leaving a tail behind.

The labelling was done with white paper cut into round shape, of the size of the lid and pasted on the lid. Labelling was done.

Viva Questions

Q. 1　What is an ointment?

Ans.　It is a solid or semisolid preparation containing medicinal ingredients in a suitable basis for external application.

Q. 2　What are the uses of sulphur ointment?

Ans.　Scabies

Q. 3　What are the uses of the ingredients of sulphur ointment.

Ans.　(i) Sulphur: It is a scabicidal. It is converted into H_2S and parathionic acid when applied to the skin. In addition to scabies, it is also employed in the treatment of other chronic skin conditions like psoriasis, ringworm.

(ii) Hard paraffin: is a mixture of solid hydrocarbons obtained from petroleum. It provides consistency to the ointment but has no medicinal value.

(iii) Wool fat: Increases the absorption of medicaments because of its hydrophillic nature. Also acts as emollient.

(iv) Soft paraffin is a simple greasy ointment which is inert chemically. It does not become rancid.

Q. 4　What are the alternative scabicidal drugs?

1. Benzyl benzoate (25%) emulsion

2. Gammexane

3. Monosulphirum

4. Crotamiton

Q. 5　How are eye ointments different from other ointments?

Ans.　1. Eye ointments have a special base: liquid paraffin 10 gm, wool fat 10 gm and white soft paraffin 80 gm.

2. Eye ointments must be free from large particles and should be prepared with aseptic precautions.

3. They should be stored in a cool place.

Q. 6　How is sulphur ointment applied?

Ans.　After a hot scrubbing soap bath, the ointment is applied from neck to foot (except scalp and face as it is irritant) for three consecutive days without any bath, followed by a soap water bath on the 4th day and all the clothings and bed sheets are washed properly.

Q. 7　What are the types of sulphur?

i. Precipitated sulphur: It is non gritty, obtained by adding HCl to a solution prepared by boiling sulphur and lime in water.

ii. Sublimed sulphur. It is gritty.

Q. 8   Write the label for this preparation.

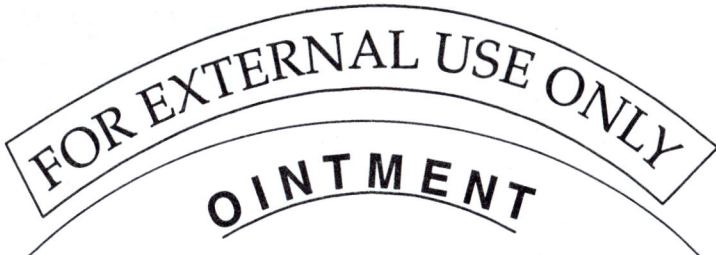

FOR EXTERNAL USE ONLY

OINTMENT

Name   : Rajeev
Age   : 25 yrs.
Regd. No. : 2156

Direction: Take a hot scrubbing bath, apply ointment on whole body below neck once daily for 3 days. Then take bath on 4th day and discard the clothes for disinfection.

UCMS Pharmacy   *Rajneesh*
25.6.04

Q. 9. Write the prescription for sulphur ointment.

Dr. Suruchi
A-5/Sec.27 RK Puram
Regd. No. 05/UCMS/416
Dated: 25-06-04

Name   : Rohit
Age   : 7 Years/Male
Regd. No. : 412

        Δ - Scabies

℞

Hard paraffin	1.35 gm
Wool fat	1.35 gm
Yellow soft paraffin	15.30 gm
Sublimed sulphur	2 gm

Direction: Mix the above and send such 20 gm.
(Apply on whole body below neck after hot scrubbing bath, once daily for 3 days.)

Suruchi
Regd. No. 05/UCMS/416

NOTES

NOTES

PART-II
Mammalian Experiments

1. RABBIT EYE

GENERAL

In the rabbit eye experiments one of these drugs is kept as the unknown drug.
1. Sympathomimetic   – Phenylephrine
2. Parasympathetic   – Physostigmine (Eserine)
3. Parasympathotytic – Atropine
4. Local anaesthetic   – Cocaine

1. Sympathomimetic

These are drugs which cause sympathetic stimulation eg. Adrenaline, Noradraneline, phenylephrine. Sympathetic stimulation cause variable effects on different systems of the body eg.

(a) Heart – Increases heart rate and force of contraction thus increasing cardiac output.

(b) Blood vessels – Vasoconstruction and increased blood pressure.

(c) Respiratory system – Bronchodilation.

(d) Gastrointestinal system and secretions – Relax smooth muscle thus ↓ peristatisis and secretions.

(e) Eye – Mydriasis by contraction of radial muscle and lower intraocular tension.

2. Parasympathomimetic Drugs

These are drugs which cause activation of parasympathetic system. Acetyl choline is the main neurotransmitter in the parasympathetic system. Acetyl choline is synthesised in local nerve endings from choline and acetyl CoA.

Choline + Acetyl CoA
↓
Acetyl Choline + CoA
↓ Ach esterase
Choline + Acetate

Acetyl choline (Ach) is inactivated with the help of the enzyme acetyl choline esterase which hydrolyses Ach to acetate and choline.

Physostigmine (trade name: Eserine) is a cholinestrase inhibitor which causes inhibition of the enzyme ach-esterase. Thus breakdown of Ach is prevented and more of ach is available to act. Therefore physotigmine acts as parasympathomimetic drug.

Parasympathomimetic drugs also have varying effects on different organs and most of the effects are antagonistic to sympathetic system. Some of these effects are:

(a) Heart - ↓ Heart Rate and force of contraction thus decreasing cardiac output.

(b) Blood vessels - Vasodilation and ↓ BP

(c) GIT - ↑ Peristalisis and secretions

(d) Respiratory system - Broncho constriction

(e) Eye - Miosis due to contraction of circular muscle of Iris and decreased intra ocular tension (i.o.t.).

3. Parasympatholytics

These are drugs which block the actions of acetyl choline. Atropine is the prototype drug of this group. It antagonises all the actions of parasympathetic system. Thus in the eye it causes mydrasis and also increases intraocular tension.

4. Local Anaesthetics:

Cocaine is a local anaesthetic which is used for ocular anaesthesia. Due to its local anaesthetic property it causes abolition of corneal reflex.

Another important property of cocaine is that it inhibits the reuptake of adrenaline and nor adrenaline into peripheral nerve endings. Reuptake is the principle mechanism by which actions of adrenaline and non adrenaline are terminated. Thus by inhibiting reuptake, cocaine causes sympathomemetic effects like local vasoconstriction, tachycardia, ↑ BP and mydriasis.

In the rabbit eye experiments four parameters are studied. These are
A. Pupil size

B. Light reflex
C. Corneal reflex
D. State of conjunctional vessels.

A. Change in Pupil Size

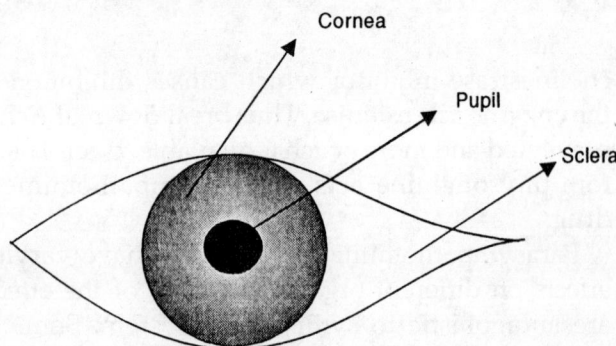

Fig. II(1)

Pupil size is controlled by two groups of muscles namely radial and circular muscles of the iris. Contraction of radial muscles (also called dilator pupillae) lead to dilatation of pupil whereas contraction of circular muscles (also called sphincter pupillae) leads to constriction of pupil.

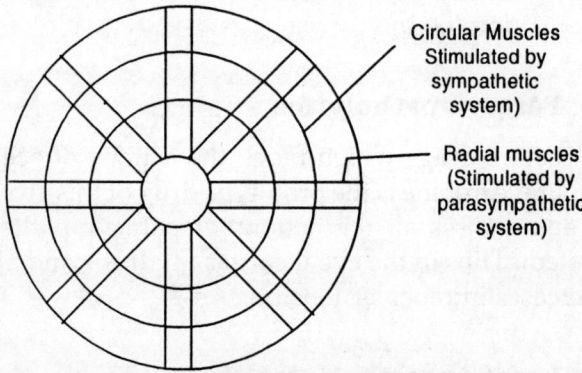

Circular Muscles
Stimulated by
sympathetic
system)

Radial muscles
(Stimulated by
parasympathetic
system)

Fig. II(2) Normal Eye

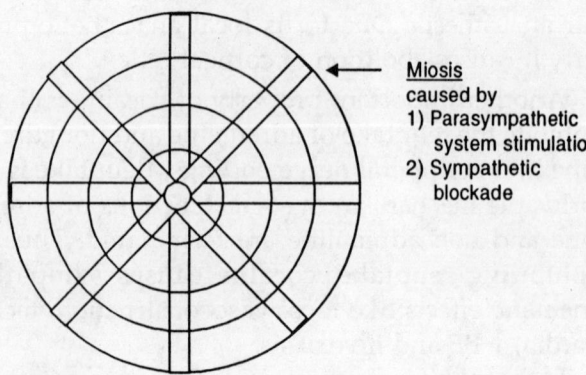

Miosis
caused by
1) Parasympathetic
system stimulation
2) Sympathetic
blockade

Fig. II(3) Contraction of sphincter pupillae and relaxation of dilator pupillae

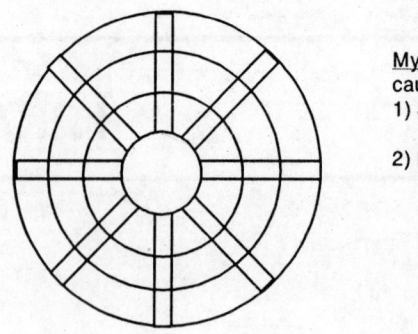

Mydriasis
caused by
1) Sympathetic
stimulation
2) Parasympathetic
blockade

Fig. II(4) Contraction of dilator pupillae and relaxation of sphincter pupillae

Active & Passive Mydriasis

1. Active mydriasis: Dilatation of pupil caused by contraction of dilator pupillae is called active mydriasis. This is caused by sympathomimetic drugs like adrenaline, phenylephrine.
2. Passive mydriasis. Dilatation of pupil caused by relaxation of constrictor pupillae is known as passive mydriasis. It is caused by parasympatholytic drugs like atropine.

Active and Passive Miosis

1. Active Miosis: Constriction of pupil caused by contraction of sphincter pupillae is called active meosis. It is caused by parasympathomimetic drugs like pilocarpine, physostigmine.
2. Passive Miosis: Constriction of pupil caused by relaxation of dilator pupilae is known as passive miosis. It is caused by sympatholytic drugs like β-blockers eg. timolol.

Effects of drugs on pupil size	
1. Phenylephrine	→ Mydriasis
2. Eserine	→ Miosis
3. Atropine	→ Mydriasis
4. Cocaine	→ Mydriasis

B. Light Reflex

Constriction of pupil on exposure to light is called light reflex.

Pathway of light reflex

Light falling on retina
↓
Optic nerve
↓
Optica chiasma
↓
Optic tract
↓
Pretectal nucleus of mid brain of both sides
↓
Edinger westphal nucleus of both sides.
↓
Oculomotor nerve (3rd cranial nerve)
↓
Ciliary ganglion (Parasympathetic ganglion)
↓
Short ciliary nerves
↓
Contraction of sphincter pupillae

There are two types of light reflex:

1. Direct light reflex: When light falls on the pupil its constriction is the direct light reflex.
2. Consensual light reflex: Impulse is relayed to both pretectal nuclei. So, when light is shed on pupil of one side, the pupil of the other side also constricts. This is the consensual light reflex.

Note: The light reflex involves only the parasympathetic system. So blockade of sympathetic system will not have any result. Blockade of the parasympathetic system will of course lead to the abolition of light reflex.

Effects of various drugs on the light reflex

Drug	Light reflex
Phenylephrine	Present
Eserine	Present
Atropine	Absent
Cocaine	Present

C. Corneal Reflex:

Closure of eye on tactile stimulation of cornea is corneal reflex.

Pathway of corneal reflex –

Tactile stimulation of cornea (with cotton swab)
↓
Trigeminal nerve (sensory nerve)
↓
Pons
↓
Facial nerve
↓
Contraction of orbularis oculi
↓
Closure of eyelid

Interruption at any point in the pathway will lead to abolition of the corneal reflex.

Local anaesthetics abolish tactile sensation of the cornea.

Effect of various drugs on the corneal reflex.

Drugs	Light reflex
Phenylephrine	Present
Eserine	Absent
Atropine	Absent
Cocaine	Absent

D. State of Conjuctival Vessels:

Conjuctiva is the outermost layer of the eyeball. It covers the sclera. The dilatation of the conjuctival vessels leads to congestion which gives the lower fornix a reddish appearance. The constriction of vessels results in a pale appearance of the lower fornix. Sympathomimetic and parasympatholytic drugs lead to constriction of vessels whereas parasympathomimetic drugs cause dilatation of the vessels.

Drug	State of conjunctival vessels
Phenylephrine	Pale
Eserine	Congested
Atropine	Pale
Cocaine	Pale

EXPERIMENT NO. 1

Aim:

To determine the effect of phenylephrine on rabbit eye.

Apparatus Required:

Rabbit, scissor, torch, cotton, pupillometer, dropper, normal saline, phenylephrine.

Procedure:

The rabbit is held in one hand in a semidark room and its eyelashes are trimmed (both eyes). Left eye serves as control and right eye as test eye. The medial canthus is pressed with one finger and with two other fingers a pouch is made for instillation of drug. Two drops of normal saline are instilled with the help of a dropper in the control (lt) eye and two drops of the drug are instilled in the test eye (Rt eye). Four parameters are measured before instillation of drug and every 5 minutes thereafter for 30 minutes. These are

1. Size of pupil
2. Light reflex
3. Corneal reflex
4. State of conjuctiva

Note: The rabbit needs to be handled very gently because frightening the rabbit may cause sympathetic stimulation leading to spurious results.

1. *Size of pupil:* It is measured with the help of a pupillometer. Increase in the size of the pupil is known as mydriasis and decrease is size is known as miosis. The size is measured is mm.

2. *Light reflex:* The light of a torch is shed on the pupil bring it from behind the eye and then moving it from lateral to medial, because if brought from the front, the rabbit may close its eyes. The contraction of the pupil on exposure to light is noted. The reaction is known as the light reflex.

3. *Corneal reflex:* A piece of cotton is taken and is rolled into a fine pointed swab and it is then touched on the lateral limbus of the rabbit eye. The closure of the eye is noticed. On touching the limbus with the swab of the eye closes it is called a positive corneal reflex.

4. *State of conjunctival vessels:* The lower eyelid of the rabbit is retracted to expose the lower palpebral conjuctiva. The vessels of the conjuctiva are observed and congestion if present is noted.

Observation:

The results are tabulated as follows:

Time:		O		5		10		15		20		25		30	
Parameter		C	T	C	T	C	T	C	T	C	T	C	T	C	T
1. Pupil size (in mm)		4	4	4	5	4	5	4	6	4	6	4	7	4	7
2. Light reflex		+	+	+	+	+	+	+	+	+	+	+	+	+	+
3. Corneal reflex		+	+	+	+	+	+	+	+	+	+	+	+	+	+
4. State of conjuctiva		Pale	Pale	Pale	Pale	Pale	Pale	Pale	Pale	Pale	Pale	Pale	Pale	Pale	Pale

Inference:

The drug phenylephrine, being a sympathomimetic increases pupil size but has no effect on light reflex, corneal reflex and state of conjuctiva.

Precautions:

1. The rabbit should be handled gently otherwise spurious results might be obtained.
2. The medical canthus should be pressed always before instilling the drug.
3. The light reflex should be tested in a semi-dark room.

Viva Questions

Q. 1 Why does the rabbit need to be gently handled in this experiment.

Ans. Because if the rabbit gets frightened, sympathetic discharge will increase leading to spurious results eg. a drug which does not cause any effect on pupil size may present as mydriatic.

Q. 2 On instilling the drug in the eye, why does the medial canthus need to be pressed?

Ans. By pressing the medial canthus, nasolacrimal duct is blocked. Thus the drug is not removed from the lacrimal sac and has more time to get absorbed. Otherwise the drug will pass through the lacrimal duct into the inferior meatus of the nose.

Q. 3 What is the mechanism of action of phenylephrine. What are its uses?

Ans. Phenylephrine is a selective α agonist. It is used for

• mydriasis when cycloplegia is not required.

• decreasing intraocular tension (by constricting the ciliary blood vessels which produce aqueous humor).

• Nasal decongestion.

Q. 4 Name one α_2 agonist and its use.

Ans. Clonidine. It is sued as anti hypertensive. By acting on presynaptic α_2 receptor it causes decreased sympathetic outflow.

Q. 5 Name β agonists and their uses.

Ans. β_1 agonist. Dobutamine used for hypo-volume shock.

β_2 agonist. Salbutanol for asthma.

Q. 6 Give the uses of adrenergic drugs.

(a) Shock, Hypovolemic - Dopamene Dobutamine

Anaphylactic, Adrenaline 0.2-0.5 mg sc.

(b) Along with local anaesthetics: Adrenaline

(c) Nasal decongestion - Phenylephrine, pseudoephedrine, rylometazoline.

(d) Cardiac arrest - Adrenaline

(e) Bronchial asthma - Slabutamol, terbutaline

(f) Mydriatic - Phenlephrine

(g) To control local bleeding like epistatis - Adrenaline

(h) Glaucoma: Depivefrine (Prodrug of adrenaline)

(i) Hyperkinetic disorder - Amphetamine

(j) An Anorectics - Fenfluramine.

Q. 7 Name some antiadrenergic drugs and their uses.

Ans.

Class of Drug	Example	Use
Selective α_1 blocker	Prazosin	Hypertension, BHP
Selective α_2 blocker	Yohimbine	Sexual disfunction
Non selective α blocker	Phenoxybenzamine	Hypertension
Selective β_1 blocker	Atenolol	Hypertension
Selective β_2 blocker	Butoxamine	
Non selective β blocker	Propanolol, Timolol	Hypertension, Glaucoma

EXPERIMENT NO. 2

Aim:

To determine the effect of atropine on rabbit eye.

Apparatus Required:

Rabbit, scissor, torch, cotton, pupillometer, dropper, normal saline, phenylephrine.

Procedure:

The rabbit is held in one hand in a semidark room and its eyelashes are trimmed (both eyes). Left eye serves as control and right eye as test eye. The medial canthus is pressed with one finger and with two other fingers a pouch is made for instillation of drug. Two drops of normal saline are instilled with the help of a dropper in the control (lt) eye and two drops of the drug are instilled in the test eye (Rt eye). Four parameters are measured before instillation of drug and every 5 minutes thereafter for 30 minutes. These are

1. Size of pupil
2. Light reflex
3. Corneal reflex
4. State of conjuctiva

Observations:

S.No.	Parameter	O C	O T	5 C	5 T	10 C	10 T	15 C	15 T	20 C	20 T	25 C	25 T	30 C	30 T
1.	Pupil size (mm)	4	4	4	5	4	5	4	6	4	6	4	7	4	7
2.	Light reflex	+	+	+	−	+	−	+	−	+	−	+	−	+	−
3.	Corneal reflex	+	+	+	+	+	+	+	+	+	+	+	+	+	+
4.	State of conjuctiva	Pale	Pale	Pale	Pale	Pale	Pale	Pale	Pale	Pale	Pale	Pale	Pale	Pale	Pale

Precautions:

1. The rabbit should be handled gently otherwise spurus results might be obtained.
2. The medical canthus should be pressed always before instilling the drug.
3. The light reflex should be test6ed in a semi-dark room.

Inference:

Atropine, being a parasympatholytic, increases pupil size and abolishes light reflex. It has no effect on corneal reflex and state of conjuctiva.

Viva Questions

Q. 1 What is the mechanism of action of atropine?
Ans. It acts via blocking the cholinergic receptors.

Q. 2 Mention the uses of atropine.
  (a) Mydriatic and cycloplegic.
  (b) Antisecretory in preanaesthetic medication
  (c) Organophosphate poisoning
  (d) As a cardiac vagolytic to counteract bradycardia.

Q. 3 Name the shortest and longest acting mydriatic.
  Shortest acting - Tropicamide
  Longest acting - Atropine

Q. 4 What are the uses of anticholinergic drugs?
  (a) Antisecretory in preanaesthetic medication eg. glycopyrolate
       Peptic ulcer - eg. Pirenzepine
  (b) Antispasmodic - eg. Hyoscine, Atropine
  (c) COPD - eg. Ipratropium, Tiotropium.
  (d) Mydriatic and cycloplegic - eg. Atropine, cyclo-pentolate, tropicamide, cycloplegic.
  (e) Motion sickness - eg. Hyoscine
  (f) Parkinsonism - eg. Trihexiphenydyl, Benztropine.
  (g) Poisonings - organophosphate poisoning - eg. Atropine

EXPERIMENT NO. 3

Aim:

To determine the effect of eserine on rabbit eye.

Apparatus:

Same as in experiment 1.

Procedure:

Same as in experiment 1.

Observations:

S.No.	Parameter	O		5		10		15		20		25		30	
		C	T	C	T	C	T	C	T	C	T	C	T	C	T
1.	Pupil size (mm)	4	4	4	3	4	3	4	2	4	2	4	1	4	1
2.	Light reflex	+	+	+	+	+	+	+	+	+	+	+	+	+	+
3.	Corneal reflex	+	+	+	+	+	+	+	+	+	+	+	+	+	+
4.	State of conjuctiva	Congested		Congested		Congested		Congested		Congested		Congested		Congested	

Inference:

Eserine a parasympathomemetic decreases pupil size and also cause congestion of conjuctiva. It has no effect on light reflex and corneal reflex.

Viva Questions

Q. 1 What is physostigmine?

Ans. It is a reversible cholinestrase inhibitor. Cholinestrase is the enzyme which is responsible for the breakdown of Ach. By blocking this enzyme, action of ach is enhanced.

Q. 2 Name some other anti cholinestrases.

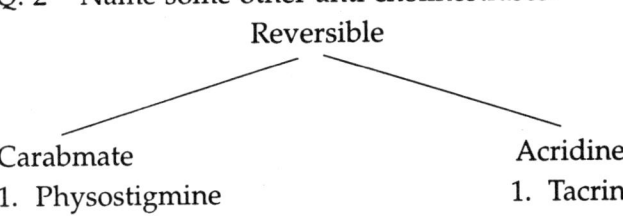

Reversible

Carabmate
1. Physostigmine
2. Neostigmine
3. Rivastigmine

Acridine
1. Tacrine

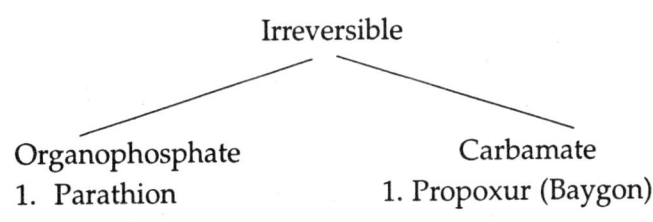

Irreversible

Organophosphate
1. Parathion
2. Malathion

Carbamate
1. Propoxur (Baygon)

Q. 3 What are the uses of anticholinestrases?

(a) Glaucoma (open angle) as miotics eg. physostimine.

(b) Paralytic ileus - eg. Neostimine

(c) Decurarization - eg. Neostigmine

(d) Cobra bite - eg. Neostigmine

(e) Myasthema gravis - eg. Neostigmine

(f) Belladona Poisoning - eg. Physostigmine

(g) Alzheimer's Disease - Tacrine, Donezepril, Revastigmine

Q. 4 What is the difference between Physostigmine and Neostigmine?

Ans. Neostigmine is a quarternary ammonium compound. So, it is not lipid soluble, and is poorly absorbed from the GIT. Also it is not able to cross the blood brain barrier or penetrate the cornea.

Physostigmine is a tertiary ammonium compound. It is rapidly absorbed from the GIT, penetrates the cornea freely and also crosses the blood brain barrier.

Due to these difference, physostigmine is used in situations where central or ocular effects are required. For example in belladona poisoning and in glaucoma. Neostigmine is preferred where central effects are not required eg. in myasthenia gravis, cobra bite etc. Also, neostigmine does not produce central side effects.

Q. 5 What is Belladona poisoning?

Ans. Belladona poisoning occurs due to ingestion of large amounts of atropa belladona, which is a source of atropine. It thus leads to anticholinergic manifestations so, the treatment is anticholinestrases like physostigmine to counteract both central peripheral effects of atropine.

Q. 6 Name the drugs used in Alzehimer's disease.

Ans. (a) Tacrine - not used now due to its hepatotoxicity.

(b) Donezepil

(c) Rivastigmene

(d) Gallantamine

Q. 7 Name the drugs used in anticholinestrase poisoning.

Ans. Atropine

Pralidoxime

Diacetylmonoxime

EXPERIMENT NO. 4

Aim:

To determine the effect of cocaine on Rabbit eye.

Apparatus:

Same as in exp. no.

Procedure:

Same as in Exp. no.

Observations:

S.No.	Parameter	O		5		10		15		20		25		30	
		C	T	C	T	C	T	C	T	C	T	C	T	C	T
1.	Pupil size (mm)	4	4	4	5	4	5	4	6	4	6	4	6	4	6
2.	Light reflex	+	+	+	+	+	+	+	+	+	+	+	+	+	+
3.	Corneal reflex	+	+	+	−	+	−	+	−	+	−	+	−	+	−
4.	State of conjuctiva	Pale	Pale	Pale	Pale	Pale	Pale	Pale	Pale	Pale	Pale	Pale	Pale		

Inference:

Cocaine being a local anaesthetic abolishes corneal reflex. Also due to its adrenergic action it causes dilation of pupil.

Precautions:

Same as in previous experiments.

Viva Questions

Q. 1   Why does cocaine cause mydriasis?

Ans.   Cocaine inhibits reuptake of adrenaline and nor adrenaline from the nerve endings. Thus it acts as a symathomimetic and causes mydriasis.

Q. 2   Why cocaine causes potentiation of action of directly acting sympathomimetics and suppression of action of indirectly acting sympathomimetics.

Ans.   Cocaine potentiates directly acting sympathomemetics as explained above. Indirectly acting sympathomimetics like tyramine are taken up by the nerve endings with the same reuptake process. After entering nerve endings these displace Adr and Noradrenaline thus causing them to enter the synapse. Thus sympathomimetus effect is produces. Since cocaine blocks reuptake process it therefore suppresses action of indirectly acting sympathomimetics.

EXPERIMENT NO. 5

Aim:

To determine the nature of unknown drug by observing its effect on Rabbit Eye.

Apparatus:

Same as in exp. 1

Procedure:

Same as in exp. 1

Observation:

The observations are noted in a table as in previous experiments.

Inference:

According to observation, the drug can be found out as.

Drug	Pupil size	Light Reflex	Corneal Reflex	State of conjuctral
Phenylephrine	↑	+	+	Pale
Eserine	↓	+	+	Congested
Atropine	↑	−	+	Pale
Cocaine	↑	−	+	Pale

Inference is written as follows:

1. If unknown drug causes mydriasis and has no effect on light & corneal reflex unknown drug is a sympathomimetic like phenylephrine.
2. If unknown drug causes miosis and has no effect on light & corneal reflex unknown drug is a parasympathomimetic like physostigmine
3. If unknown drug causes mydriasis and abolition of light reflex unknown drug is parasympatholytic like atropine
4. If unknown drug causes mydriosis and abolition of corneal reflex unknown drug is cocaine

NOTES

NOTES

2. RABBIT ILEUM

GENERAL

A. APPARATUS

(1) Dale's Organ Bath: This apparatus consists of following parts [Fig. II(5)]:

    (a) Rectangular Bath: It is made up of perspex. It contains a glass tube in the centre and also contains a heating element, a thermostat and stirrer. Water is added in the outer bath and heated with heating element and kept at about 37°C with the help of a thermostat. 3-4 test tubes containing ringer solution are kept in outer bath to keep the temperature of ringer near 37°C.

    (b) Inner Bath: It is a central glass organ bath and is provided with an outlet. Its capacity is 20ml. Through the outlet, ringer is removed while washing the tissue. A bent glass tube is placed in the inner bath.

    (c) Bent glass tube: It is hollow and curved at the lower end. The curved end is used to tie the rabbit ileum. Oxygen is provided to the tissue through it.

    (d) Frontal writing lever [Fig. II(7)]: The other end of the ileum is attached to frontal writing lever with the help of a thread. A pen marker is attached to frontal writing lever for recording the contractions.

    (e) Heating Element: It is used for heating the water in outer bath.

    (f) Thermostat: It keeps the temperature nearly constant at about 37°C.

    (g) Side Rods: Two metallic side rods are attached to the rectangular bath. One is used to fix the bent glass tube and the other is used to fix the frontal writing lever.

(2) Aeration Tube: A rubber tubing is attached to the air bubbler for providing oxygen. Oxygen also helps in mixing the drug in the solution.

(3) Petri Dish: It is used to keep the isolated ileum while fixing the threads on both its ends.

(4) Thermometer: A thermometer is kept in outer bath to check the temperature.

(5) Kymograph [Fig. II(6)]: It is used to record the movements on a moving surface. It has the following parts

    (a) Electric Motor: It helps to rotate the shift and drum. It operates at 220 volts AC.

    (b) Shaft: It is connected to the motor vertically. Shaft can be made to rotate at various speeds ranging from 0.25 mm/sec to 640 mm/sec.

    (c) Drum: It is 15 cm × 15 cm cylinder which is mounted on the shaft. Drum rotates when the shaft rotates. A white paper is pasted on the drum. On the shaft, there is drum grip lever, which helps in locking and unlocking of drum. The level of drum can be adjusted as desired.

    (d) Gears: These are used for changing the speed of the drum. Speed of drum can be adjusted from 0.25 mm/sec (minimum) to 640 mm/sec (maximum).

    (e) Clutch: This is used to start or stop the rotation of drum. It disengages the gear from axle of the motor. It must be used everytime before changing the gears.

    (f) Levelling Screws: Two levelling screws are present at the base which help in proper levelling of the instrument in a horizontal plane.

B. Principle

It is based on the principle that when isolated piece of rabbit's intestine is placed into similar environment as that of extra cellular fluid, it shows the property of auto-rythmicity and the effect of various drugs can be studied on it.

C. Theory

One of the following five drugs is given in this

experiment and this drug has to be identified. These drugs are

1. Acetylcholine
2. Adrenaline
3. Papaverine
4. Barium chloride
5. Atropine

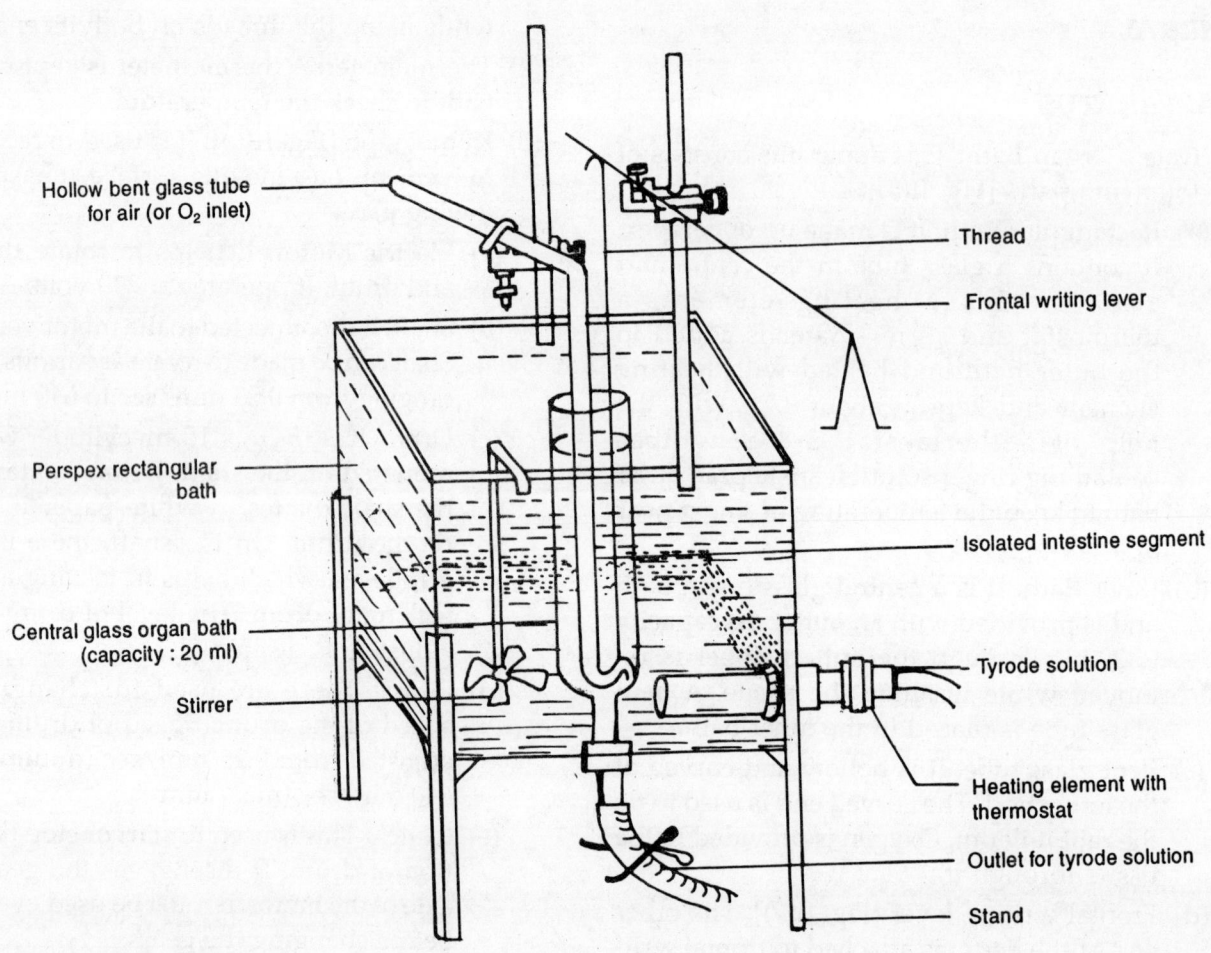

Hollow bent glass tube for air (or O₂ inlet)

Thread

Frontal writing lever

Perspex rectangular bath

Isolated intestine segment

Central glass organ bath (capacity : 20 ml)

Tyrode solution

Stirrer

Heating element with thermostat

Outlet for tyrode solution

Stand

Fig. II(5) *Dale's Organ Bath*

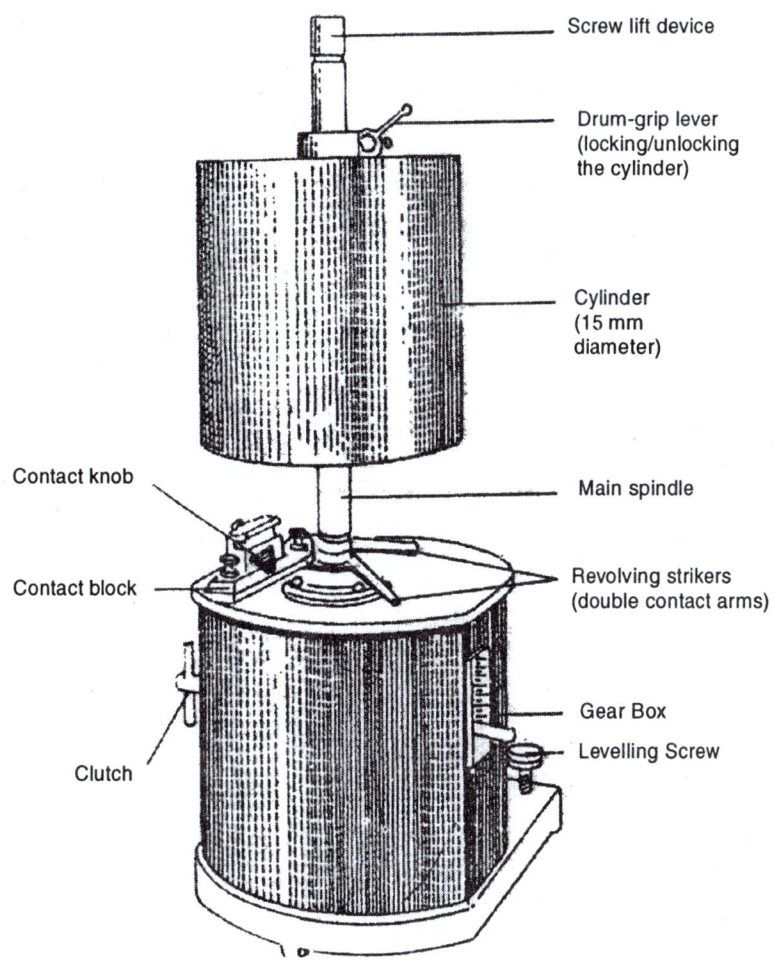

Screw lift device

Drum-grip lever
(locking/unlocking
the cylinder)

Cylinder
(15 mm
diameter)

Contact knob

Main spindle

Contact block

Revolving strikers
(double contact arms)

Gear Box

Levelling Screw

Clutch

Fig. II(6) *Kymograph*

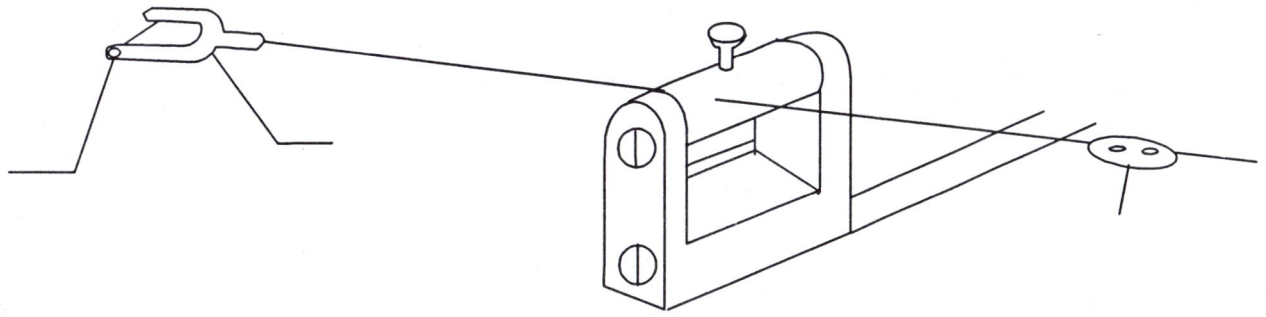

Fig. II(7) *Frontal Writing Lever*

EXPERIMENT NO.1

Aim:

To study the effect of acetylcholine on isolated rabbit's ileum.

Requirements:

Kymograph, petridish, isolated organ bath (Dale's organ bath), frontal writing lever, ink writing recorder, air bubbler connected with aeration tube, tuberculin syringe, tyrode's ringer solution, thermometer, hot plate to make hot water for isolated organ bath, plasticene, rabbit ileum, acetylcholine chloride (1:10,000).

Procedure:

1. Kymograph is adjusted to rotate at a speed of 0.25 mm/sec. and the lever is balanced with a magnification factor of 5.
2. A 3-4 cm long piece of ileum or jejunum is taken in a porcelain petri dish containing tyrode's solution. Lumen of the loop of intestine is cleaned by pushing gently the tyrode's solution with the help of a syringe.
3. A loop of thread is tied at one end without occluding the lumen and another thread is tied at diametrically opposite end.
4. Inner organ bath is filled with tyrode's solution and outer bath is filled with warm water maintained at 37°C. A thermometer is kept in the outer bath to check the maintenance of temperature.
5. One end of the intestine is tied to the S-shaped part of aeration tube. it is then immersed in tyrode's solution present in the inner bath. Other end of the intestine is tied to short arm of frontal writing lever . Small amount of extra plasticene is added on the long arm to stretch the intestine.

   Flow of oxygen through the aeration tube is adjusted to provide a constant flow. Care is taken that the thread and the piece of intestine don't touch the side walls of bath. The volume of inner bath is marked and kept constant.
6. Three or four test tubes filled with tyrode solution should be kept immersed in outer bath so that the temperature of tyrode's solution in-

creases to 37°C. These are used for changing the fluid in the inner bath.
7. Pen marker is attached to the kymograph drum, on which paper has been pasted. Normal contractions are then recorded.
8. Then 0.1 ml of drug solution (1:10,000 acetylcholine) is instilled in the inner bath and contractions are recorded for 30 seconds. If the effect produced is not very prominent, the dose of drug should be doubled. The procedure is repeated after washing.

Observations:

1. The tracing from kymograph is pasted on the practical file.

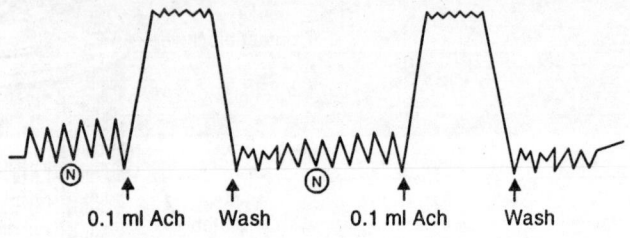

0.1 ml Ach   Wash   0.1 ml Ach   Wash

Fig. II(8)

2. From the kymograph tracing it is noted that on adding 0.1 ml Ach (1:10,000), there is

   • increase in tone
   • decrease in amplitude
   • increase in frequency

Inference:

As ACh increases the tone and frequency of ileal contractions, it acts as a stimulant drug. The decrease of amplitude is secondary to increased tone.

Precautions:

1. Ileum should not be injured or mishandled.
2. The temperature of tyrode's solution should be kept at 37°C and it should be properly aerated.
3. Lumen of the intestine should not be blocked.
4. Threads are tied to the opposite ends of the ileum without obstructing the lumen.
5. Thread or intestine should not touch the side walls of inner bath.

Viva Questions

Q. 1. What is the composition and function of tyrode's solution?

Ans. Tyrode's solution is used for isolated mammalian tissues. It is also called mammalian ringer solution. Its composition is

Glucose	- 1g
NaCl	- 0.8g
KCl	- 0.2g
$CaCl_2$	- 0.2g
$MgCl_2$	- 0.1g
$NaHCl_3$	- 0.1g
NaH_2PO_4	- 0.05g
Aqua ad	- 1 litre

The functions of ingredients are
1. Glucose: provides nutrition
2. NaCl, KCl, $CaCl_2$:
   a. helps to maintain isotonicity
   b. electrical neutrality is maintained
3. $NaHCO_3$, NaH_2PO_4: helps to maintain pH between 7.4 to 7.6
4. $MgCl_2$: helps to regulate intestinal motility.

Q. 2. What is the capacity of inner organ bath?

Ans. 20 ml

Q. 3. What is the use of aeration?

Ans. 1. It provides oxygen to the ileum.
2. It helps in mixing of the drug.

Q. 4. What is the mechanism of action of Ach?

Ans. Acetylcholine acts on the muscarinic (M_3) receptors in the intestine and stimulates the intestinal contractions by increasing Na^+ and Ca^{2+} influx.

Q. 5. How do you explain the decrease in amplitude of intestinal contractions by Ach?

Ans. Because of increase in basal tone of intestinal smooth muscle by acetylcholine, it is not able to contract more forcefully, resulting in decrease in amplitude.

Q. 6. What are other stimulant drugs of intestine?

Ans. 1. Para sympathomimetics –
      Acetylcholine
      Carbachol
      Anticholinesterases
2. Sympatholytics β-Blockers
3. Calcium chloride ($CaCl_2$)
4. Barium chloride ($BaCl_2$)
5. Histamine - It is a (direct stimulant of GIT, and also facilitates the action of ACh)

Q. 7. What are the therapeutic uses of smooth muscle stimulants?

Ans. 1. Post operative paralytic ileus: e.g. Neostigmine
2. Post operative urinary retention: e.g. Neostigmine

Q. 8. Why is the duration of action of Ach shorter than that of carbachol ?

Ans. Both of these drugs are cholinergic agonists. Acetylcholine is degraded by both acetylcholine esterase and butrylcholine esterase, so its duration of action is very short, on the other hand carbachol is not metabolized by these enzymes, so its duration of action is longer.

Q. 9. Why is d-Tubocurarine used as a blocker of action of acetylcholine in frog rectus preparation whereas atropine is used for the same function in rabbit ileum experiment?

Ans. At skeletal muscle junction, there are nicotinic receptors, the blocker of which is d-Tubocurarine. So, in frog rectus muscle (a skeletal muscle), dTC is used as a blocker.

In smooth muscles, (rabbit ileum) muscarinic receptors are present and atropine is a blocker of muscarinic receptors. Therefore, atropine is used as a blocker in rabbit ileum experiments.

EXPERIMENT NO. 2

Aim:

To study the effect of adrenaline on isolated rabbit's ileum.

Requirements:

Same as in Exp. No. 1 except that adrenaline (1:10,000) is required in place of acetylcholine.

Procedure:

1. Set up of apparatus and mounting of tissue is done as in Experiment No. 1.
2. Normal tracing is taken and then 0.1 ml of adrenaline (1:10,000) is added to inner bath.
3. Tracing is recorded and if the response is not adequate, dose is doubled till the acceptable response occurs.
4. After washing, the drug is confirmed by adding the same amount.

Observations:

1. Kymograph Tracings

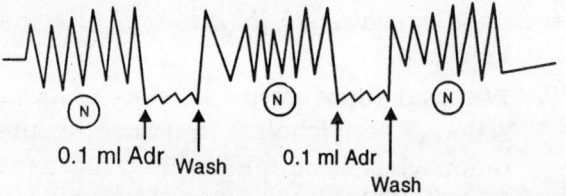

Fig. II(9)

2. From the tracing, it is clear that on adding adrenaline,
   (a) Frequency decreases
   (b) Tone decreases
   (c) Amplitude decreases

Inference:

Adrenaline is a sympathomimetic drug and it depresses the rabbit ileal smooth muscle.

Precautions:

Same as Experiment No. 1

Viva Questions

Q. 1. What is the mechanism of action of adrenaline on smooth muscle of intestine?

Ans. Adrenaline acts on α and β adrenergic receptors in the intestine. β-effect is mediated through cAMP and α-effect is mediated through Ca^{2+} efflux via these mechanisms, adrenaline depress intestinal contractions.

Q. 2. What are antispasmodics or spasmolytics of GIT?

Ans. Antispasmodics reduce the intestinal spasms i.e. depress the contractions. These are classified as
   (a) Sympathomimetics: Adrenaline, Isoprenaline
   (b) Anti-Cholinergics: Atropine
   (c) Ganglion Blockers: Hexamethonim
   (d) Directly Acting: Papaverine, Xanthines, Nitrites

Q. 3. What are the therapeutic uses of Antispasmodics?

Ans. 1. Intestinal colic: Atropine, Hyoscine
   2. Ureteric colic: Atropine, Hyoscine
   3. Biliary colic: Papaverine, Nitrites
   4. Bronchal Asthma: Aminophylline

Q. 4. How do you block the action of adrenaline on intestinal smooth muscles?

Ans. We can block the action of adrenaline by giving both α-receptor antagonist and β-blocker.

EXPERIMENT NO. 3

Aim:

To study the effect of Barium chloride on isolated rabbit ileum.

Requirements:

Same as in Experiment No. 1 plus adrenaline (1:10,000) and Barium chloride (1%)

Procedure:

1. Set up and mounting of tissue is done as in

Experiment No.1

2. Normal recording is taken and then 0.1 ml of acetylcholine solution (1:10,000) is added. Recording is taken for 30s and then washing of the drug is done. Then 0.1 ml of adrenaline solution (1:10,000) is added and recording is again taken for 30s. These drugs are added to check the sensitivity of the tissue to known stimulant and depressant.

3. After washing, 0.1ml of $BaCl_2$ is added and the recording is taken. If no visible effect is present, double the dose is added till the effect become visible.

Observations:

(1) Kymograph Tracing

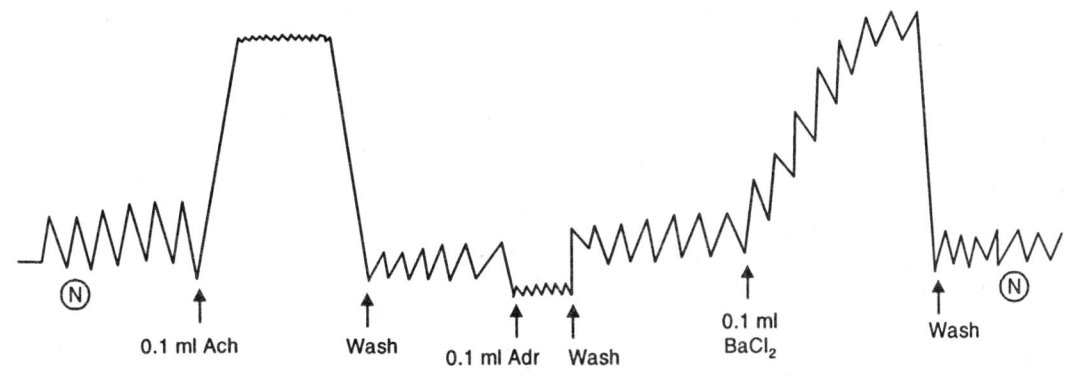

Fig. II(10)

(2) From the Kymograph Tracing, it is clear that

 – rabbit ileum is sensitive to Ach and adrenaline
 – $BaCl_2$ increases the tone, frequency and amplitude of contractions.

Inference:

Barium chloride has a stimulant action on the smooth muscle of ileum.

Precautions:

The sensitivity testing must be done first with stimulant drug (ACh) and then with depressant drug (Adrenaline). The rest of precautions are the same as in Experiment No. 1.

Viva Questions

Q. 1   What is the mechanism of action of barium chloride on rabbit ileal smooth muscle?

Ans.   It is a directly acting drug which stimulates smooth muscles directly.

Q. 2   Where is Barium used?

Ans.   1. $BaCl_2$ is used as a rat poison because it stimulates the intestines and produces violent colicky pain.
2. $BaSO_4$ is used in radiographic studies like
  – Barium swallow
  – Barium meal
  – Barium follow through
  – Barium enema

Q. 3   What are the various radiographic studies in which barium is used?

Ans. (a) *Barium Swallow*: a paste of barium is given to swallow and radiographs (X rays) are taken. It is used to study the lesions of pharynx and esophagus.

(b) *Barium Meal*: Delayed radiographs are taken after giving barium by mouth. It is used for the study of lesions involving stomach and proximal small intestines.

(c) *Barium Follow Through*: After giving barium sulphate by mouth, radiographs are taken after 4-6 hours to visualise intestines.

(d) *Barium Enema*: In this investigation barium sulphate is instilled per rectally and radiographs are taken to visualise rectum and sigmoid colon.

Q. 4 Is the action of $BaCl_2$ on rabbit ileum similar to that due to ACh?

Ans. Both ACh and $BaCl_2$ have stimulant action on rabbit ileum but the action is not exactly similar. In case of acetylcholine, there is immediate rise of tone and frequency but in case of $BaCl_2$, there is gradual increase in tone and amplitude, (staircase phenomenon).

Q. 5. Why is $BaSO_4$ used in barium meal rather than $BaCl_2$?

Ans. $BaSO_4$ is insoluble in water and thus is not absorbed whereas $BaCl_2$ is soluble and gets absorbed. Due to this reason $BaCl_2$ causes poisoning and $BaSO_4$ does not.

Q. 6. How will you differentiate the action of $BaCl_2$ and ACh?

Ans. 1. **By the nature of effect produced.** $BaCl_2$ produces staircase phenomenon whereas ACh produces sudden rise of tone and frequency.

2. **On giving atropine**, effect of ACh is blocked but not that of $BaCl_2$.

EXPERIMENT NO. 4

Aim:

To study the effect of papaverine on isolated rabbit ileum.

Requirements:

Same as in Experiment No.1 plus adrenaline (1:10,000) and papaverine (0.1%).

Observations:

1. Kymograph Tracing

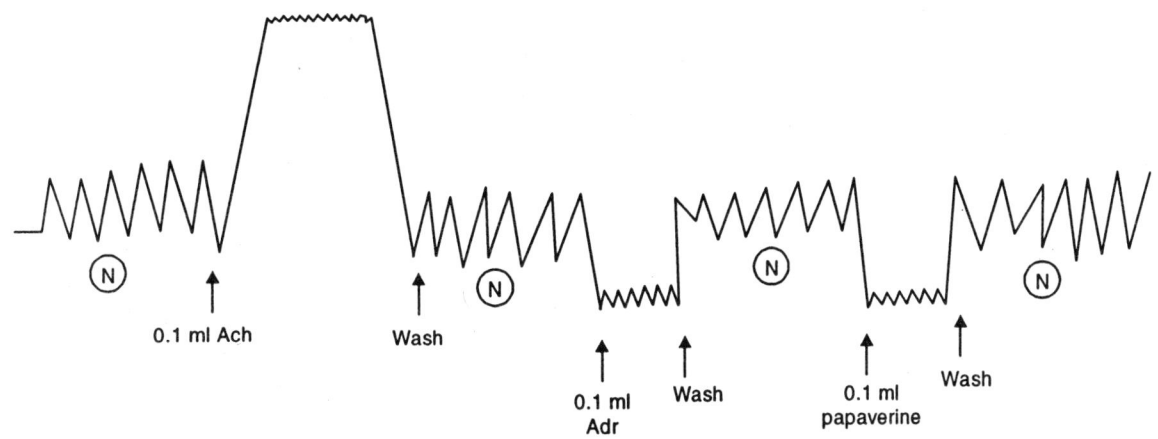

Fig. II(11)

Procedure:

1. Set up and mounting of tissue is done as in Experiment No.1.
2. Sensitivity of ileum is tested to ACh and adrenaline as in Experiment No. 3.
3. After recording the baseline, 0.1 ml of papaverine hydrochloride (0.1%) is instilled in the inner organ bath and tracing is taken.

2. From the Kymograph Tracing, it is clear that
   – tissue is sensitive to Ach & Adr
   – papaverine produces decrease in amplitude, frequency and tone of contractions

Inference:

Papaverine produces depression in rabbit ileal activity i.e. acts as smooth muscle relaxer.

Precautions:

Same as in Experiment No. 3.

Viva Questions

Q. 1. What is the mechanism of action of papaverine on rabbit's ileum?

Ans. Papaverine produces relaxation of rabbit ileal smooth muscle by acting directly.

Q. 2. How will you differentiate that the given relaxant is papaverine and not adrenaline?

Ans. On giving both α and β receptor blockers, there is absence of depressor action of adrenaline whereas papaverine retains its relaxant property even after giving blockers.

Q. 3. Name other relaxants of smooth muscles?

Ans. Adrenaline

Atropine

Q. 4. To which group does papaverine belong?

Ans. Papaverine is a natural opioid alkaloid.

Q. 5. What are the uses of papaverine?

Ans. Papaverine acts as a smooth muscle relaxant thus it can be used in

– Biliary colic as antispasmodic.

– PIPE (Papaverine Induced Penile Erection) therapy for impotence.

EXPERIMENT NO. 5

Aim:

To study the effect of atropine on isolated rabbit ileum.

Requirements:

Same as in Experiment No. 1 and also 1:10,000 adrenaline solution and 1:10,000 atropine sulphate solution.

Observations:

1. Kymograph Tracing

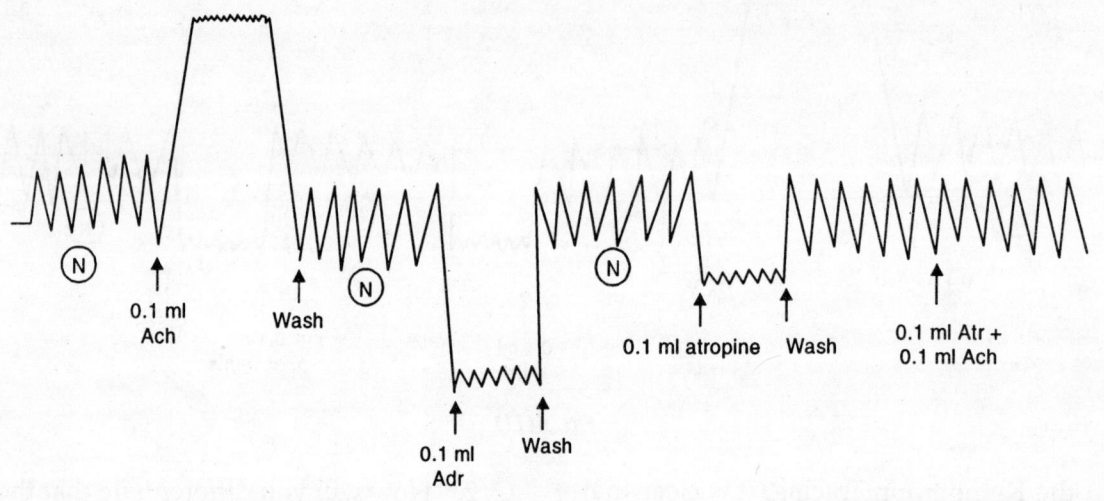

Fig. II(12)

Procedure:

1. Set up and mounting of tissue is done as in Experiment No. 1.
2. Sensitivity of the tissue is checked as in Experiment No. 3.
3. After taking base line tracing, 0.1 ml of atropine (1:10,000) is added to the inner bath and recording is taken.
4. After washing, recording is taken again to confirm the action and then 0.1 ml Ach is added two minutes after adding atropine.

2. From the kymograph tracing, it is observed that
   (1) Tissue is sensitive to acetylcholine and adrenaline.
   (2) On adding atropine, there is relaxation of intestinal smooth muscle.
   (3) Atropine blocks the stimulant action of Ach.

Inference:

Atropine relaxes the intestinal smooth muscle by blocking the action of acetylcholine.

Precautions:

It is advised to wait for two minutes after adding atropine and only then Ach should be added (without washing). The rest of precautions are same as before.

Viva Questions

Q. 1 What is the mechanism of action of atropine on rabbit ileal smooth muscle?

Ans. Atropine is a muscarinic receptor blocker and it blocks the stimulant effect of Ach on muscarinic receptors in intestinal smooth muscles.

Q. 2 If there is no effect of atropine on rabbit ileum, what does it signify?

Ans. Atropine itself produces no effect on rabbit ileal smooth muscle. Instead, it inhibits the action of acetylcholine on muscarinic receptors in ileal smooth muscles. If the resting activity of parasympathetic system is low, there will be no appreciable effect of atropine. But atropine will always block the stimulant action of acetylcholine.

Q. 3 What are the uses of atropine as an antispasmodic?

Ans. It can be used to relieve intestinal and biliary colics.

Q. 4 What are the other uses of atropine?

Ans. Atropine can also be used as
  – Mydriatic in children
  – Antidote for organophosphate and carbamate poisoning.

Q. 5 What is the absolute contra indication for the use of atropine?

Ans. Narrow angle glaucoma

Q. 6 Before adding acetylcholine in this experiment it is advised to wait for two minutes after atropine addition. Why?

Ans. Two minutes are given for atropine to block all the muscarinic receptors present in intestinal smooth muscle.

EXPERIMENT NO. 6

Aim:

To determine the nature of unknown drug by studying its effect on isolated rabbit ileum.

Requirements:

- 1:10,000 Ach Solution
- 1:10,000 Atropine Solution
- 1:10,000 Adrenaline Solution
- 1:10,000 Propanolol solution (β-Blocker)

The rest is same as in Experiment No. 1.

Procedure:

1. Set up and mounting of tissue is done as in Experiment No. 1.
2. Sensitivity of the tissue to Ach and Adr is checked as in Experiment No. 3.
3. After taking normal tracing for 30 s, 0.1 ml of unknown drug is added and its effect is studied. It can be

   A. Stimulant – Acetylcholine or $BaCl_2$
   B. Depressant – Adrenaline, papverine, atropine
   C. No Effect – Atropine.

If the Unknown Drug is Stimulant: If the unknown drug increases the tone, frequency or amplitude of contractions, then the experiment is proceeded as follows

- Drug is washed and 0.2 ml of atropine solution is added.
- After waiting for 2 minutes and without washing, same amount of unknown drug is again added.
- If the stimulant effect of Ach is abolished, the unknown drug must be para-sympathomimetic like acetylcholine and if the stimulant effect still persists, it must be acting directly like $BaCl_2$ or histamine.

If the Unknown Drug is Depressant:

If the unknown drug produces relaxation, then it may be atropine, adrenaline or papaverine. Now the experiment is proceeded as follows:-

- Without washing unknown drug, 0.1 ml of ACh is added to inner organ bath. If the stimulant effect of acetylcholine is not present, then it must be parasympatholytic drug like atropine. If the stimulant effect of ACh persists, then proceed to next step.
- After washing record a baseline tracing and then add 0.2 ml of β-Blocker like propanolol.
- After waiting for 2 minutes, add 0.1 ml of unknown drug and obtain the tracing. If the depressant effect of unknown drug abolishes, then it must be sympathomi-metic drug like adrenaline. If the depressant effect of unknown drug still persists, and with same magnitude, then unknown drug must be a directly acting depressant like papaverine.

If Unknown Drug Produces No Effect:

If there is no effect of unknown drug, then dose is doubled to 0.2 ml. If still no response occurs, then 0.4 ml dose is used. Even then if no response occurs, then without washing 0.1 ml of Ach is added. The stimulant effect of acetylcholine abolishes and thus unknown drug must be parasympatholytic like atropine.

Inference:

Inference should be written as follows:-
The unknown drug is.......................
(sympathomimetic/Parasympatho-mimetic/Parasympatholytic/Directly acting stimulant/Directly acting depressant, as the case may be.)

Precautions:

Same as in Experiment No. 5.

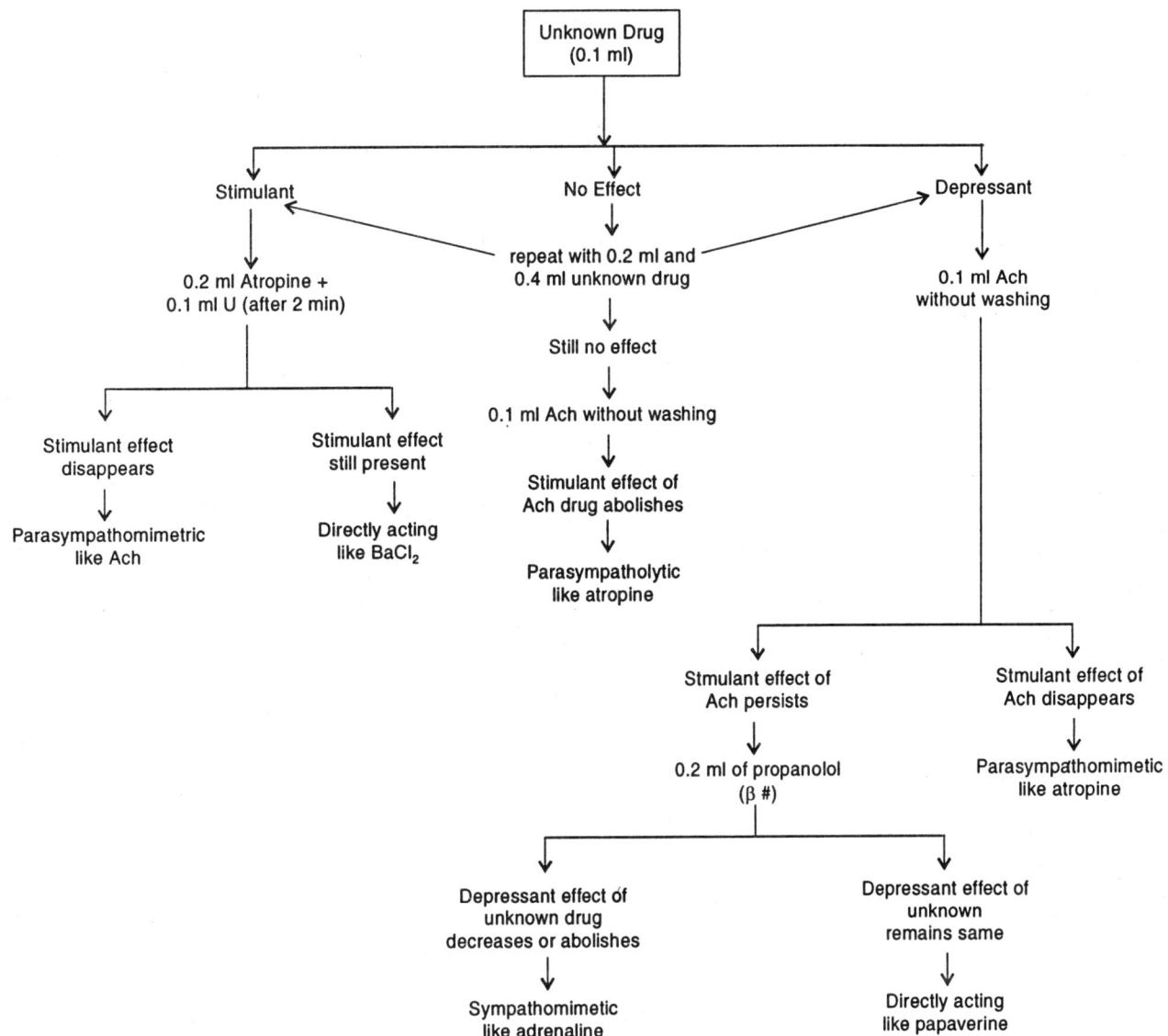

Viva Questions

Q. 1 What is the function of aeration tube and air bubbler?

Ans. These perform two important functions:
1. To oxygenate the tissue.
2. Help in mixing of the drug in the ringer solution.

Q. 2 In frog's rectus abdominis muscle, extra weights are required to relax the muscle but in the rabbit ileum experiment the muscle is not relaxed by using extra-weights. Why?

Ans. Frog's rectus abdominis muscle is a slow contracting muscle, so it requires extraweights to be kept for about 30 min. In case of rabbit ileum, the muscle is fast contracting and fast relaxing. So extraweights are not required to relax the muscle.

Q. 3 What is the importance of studying drug actions on "smooth muscle preparations"?

Ans. These type of studies are important because smooth muscle is found in practically all internal organs like gastro-intestinal tract, bronchial muscle, urinary tract, bile duct, uterus etc. Further, the pharmacological actions of these drugs are similar on all these organs except uterus.

Q. 4 Why have you chosen isolated rabbit ileum for your study?

Ans. We have chosen isolated rabbit ileum as it is quite convenient to mount this tissue in an isolated organ bath and study the effect of drugs on either their spontaneous motility or drug induced spasms.

Q. 5 What is the nerve supply of smooth muscles?

Ans. Smooth muscles are supplied by both divisions of Autonomic Nervous System i.e. sympathetic and parasympathetic. These usually operate in opposite directions.

Q. 6 What are different types of movements of intestine?

Ans. There are three main types of intestinal movements.

A. *Pendular Movements*: These help in propagation and churning of food. These movements are performed by Longitudinal muscle fibres.

B. *Segmental Movements:* These helps in churning of food. These are performed by circular muscle fibres.

C. *Peristaltic or Propulsive Movements:* These movements help mainly in propagation of food. These are due to both circular and longitudinal muscle fibres.

Q. 7 Which type of movements are you recording in your experiment?

Ans. In this experiment, composite movements are recorded. These are mainly pendular and slightly segmental. Peristaltic movements cannot be recorded in vitro.

Q. 8 Why is water kept in the outer bath in this experiment and not in frog's rectus abdominus muscle experiment?

Ans. Frog is a cold blooded animal and does not require strict maintenance of temperature for its functioning. Rabbit is a warm blooded animal and its tissues require temperature of about 37°C for their functioning. Water is added in the outer bath and heated to keep the temperature of the ringer solution in the inner bath at about 37°C. Therefore water is added in outer bath in rabbit's isolated organ experiments and not in frog's isolated organ experiments.

Q. 9 What will happen if lumen of intestinal segment is obstructed?

Ans. Lumen obstruction will cause the contractions to disappear.

Q. 10 Why is extra plasticene added to the long arm of lever?

Ans. By adding extra plasticene, there is longitudinal stretching of isolated segment of intestine. Longitudinal stretching results in increase in tone and amplitude of contractions. However, optimal length produces maximum response and stretching beyond an optimal length produces opposite effect.

Q. 11 What is the effect of histamine on isolated rabbit ileal muscle. What is its mechanism?

Ans. Histamine has stimulating effect on isolated rabbit ileal smooth muscle. It increases the frequency of contractions. It produces stimulation by two mechanisms.

1. It has direct stimulatory effect on smooth muscles.

2. It also facilitates the action of Ach.

Q. 12 On adding β-blocker, there is complete abolition of effect of adrenaline on frog heart experiment whereas the response is reduced and not fully abolished on adding β-Blocker in isolated rabbit ileum experiment. Why?

Ans. In heart, there are mainly β_1 receptors and adrenaline acts on these receptors to produce stimulation. So by blocking the action of these receptors, β-adrenergic antagonists abolishes this effect. On the other hand, both α and β receptors mediate the relaxation of ileal smooth muscle. Adrenaline acts on both of these receptors to produce relaxation. On adding β-adrenergic antagonists only β-mediated relaxation is abolished but α-receptor mediated relaxation persists. Therefore relaxing response of adrenaline is only partly reversed on addition of β-blocker.

NOTES

NOTES

PART-III
Amphibian Experiments

1. FROG HEART

GENERAL

Apparatus:

1. *Kymograph:* It is used for recording the graph and is explained in experiment on Rabbit Ileum. [Fig. II(6)]

2. *Marriote Bottle* [Fig. III(1)]: It is an ordinary bottle with a side opening near the bottom. Its mouth is fitted with a tight cork through which a glass tube is passed and the tube reaches nearly upto the bottom. The bottle is named after a french physiologist, Mariotte. It is used as a reservoir of frog ringer. During perfusion experiments, the perfusion fluid should profuse the organ at a constant pressure so that a constant amount of fluid can perfuse the organ. Its advantage is that, with this bottle a steady pressure head can be maintained.

3. *Perfusion Apparatus:* It consists of the Mariotte bottle, rubber tubing and a venous cannula. Rubber tubing is connected to the perfusion bulb on one end and to the venous cannula on the other end. Venous cannula is inserted in the inferior vena cava and the ringer is supplied via this perfusion apparatus.

4. *Frontal Writing Lever* [Fig. III(2)]: It is type I isotonic lever [fulcrum lies between the writing point and site of attachment of tissue]. To one end of this lever, frog heart is attached via a thread and to the other end ink writing recorder is attached. It writes frontally and perpendicular to the drum.

Theory:

In the examination, one of five drugs will be given and student has to identify the nature of unknown drug by its effect of frog heart. The drugs that will be given are:

1. Adrenaline

2. Acetylcholine

3. Calcium chloride

4. Potassium chloride

5. Atropine

Heart is innervated by both divisions of autonomic nervous system i.e. sympathetic as well as parasympathetic. Sympathetic system causes stimulation of heart i.e. increase in force of contraction (amplitude), increase in rate (decreased distance in tracing) and increase in tone (raised baseline). Parasympathetic system stimulation causes decrease in amplitude, rate and tone. Adrenaline is a sympathomimetic drug and acetylcholine is a parasympathomimetic drug. Atropine blocks muscarinic cholinergic receptors and thus acts as parasymapatholytic. Calcium chloride is directly acting stimulant whereas potassium chloride is directly acting depressant drug.

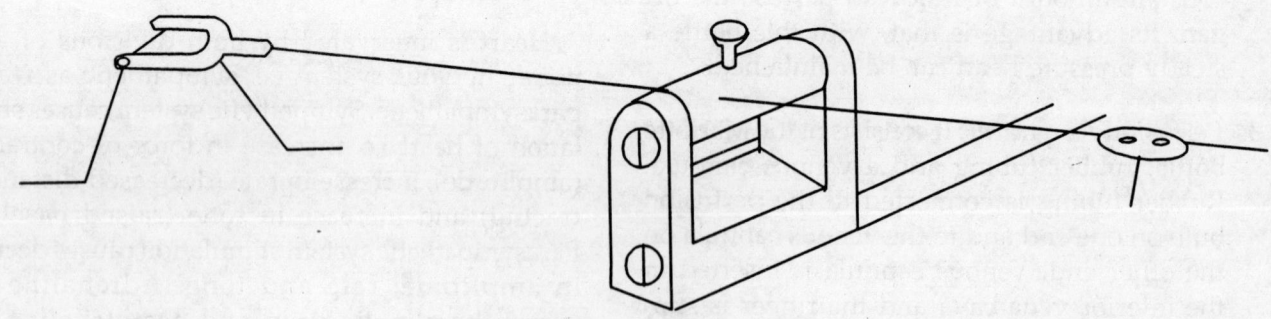

Fig. III(1). Mariotte Bottle

Fig. III(2) Frontal Writing Lever

(a)

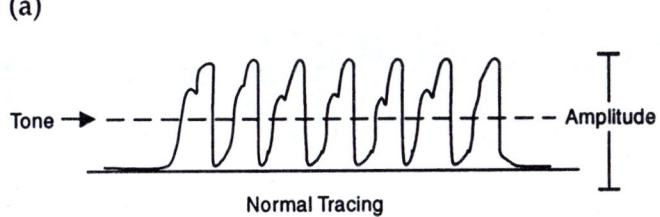

Fig. III(3)

(b)

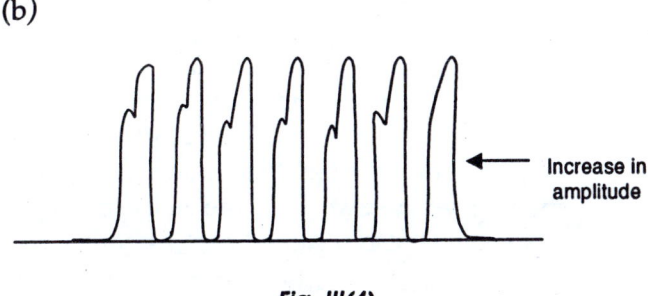

Fig. III(4)

(c)

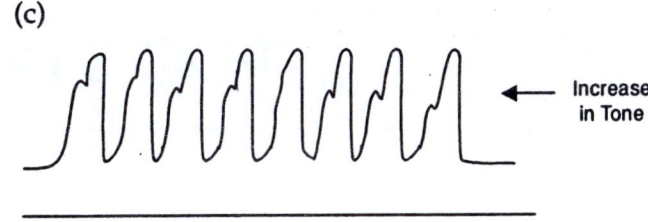

Fig. III(5)

(d)

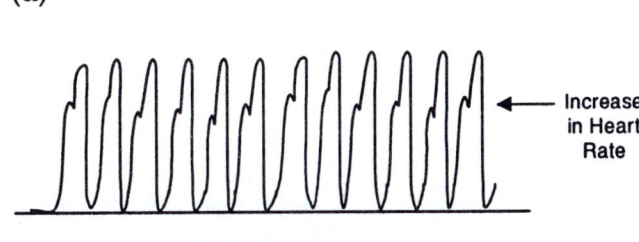

Fig. III(6)

Observations:

Following are observed in the tracing before and after adding adrenaline.

(i) *Amplitude of Contraction:* It is the total height of tracing. Increase in amplitude means forceful contraction and stimulation and decrease in amplitude of contraction means depression.

(ii) *Cardiac Tone:* Increase in the tone is indicated by the upward shift of baseline while decrease is indicated by downward shift of base line.

(iii) *Cardiac Rate:* Increase of heart rate is indicated by contraction coming close to each other and decrease of heart rate is shown by contractions being far apart.

2. FROG'S PERFUSED HEART

EXPERIMENT NO. 1

Aim:

To study the effect of Adrenaline on perfused frog's heart is situ.

Requirements:

Kymograph, frog board, dissection set, perfusion apparatus (perfusion bulb fitted with cork and glass tube, rubber tubing, venous cannula, retort stand with a ring for holding the perfusion bulb), iron stand, frontal writing lever, thread, pins, tuberculin syringe, pithing needle, frog's ringer solution, adrenaline (1:100,000) and frog.

Procedure:

(1) A paper is pasted on the drum of kymograph and it is set ready to rotate at a speed of 0.25 mm/s. The lever is balanced and perfusion apparatus is set up using frog's ringer solution. All air bubbles are removed from the rubber tubing and cannula.

(2) *Dissection of the frog:*

   (a) A big frog is taken. It is stunned with the help of a hammer. A pithing needle is inserted in the spinal cord towards the cephalic end and brain is destroyed. Then direction of the needle is reversed and spinal cord is destroyed. Pithing is complete when there is extension of all four limbs. Now, the frog is placed on the frog board with back down and pinned on it. Skin is slit open. The abdominal wall is removed by a V-shaped incison from pelvis to pectoral girdle. The pericardium is now slit open to expose the heart and a few drops of ringer are poured over the heart.

   (b) A pin is bent and this bent pin is inserted through the ventricular apex as a hook. With the pin and the thread attached to it, the heart is pulled anteriorly.

   (c) Inferior vena cava is now identified and cleared upto hepatic veins. Two threads are passed underneath it. A V-shaped nick is made in the inferior vena cava in the direction of heart. A venous cannula is taken from which all air has been expelled and this cannula is now inserted in the inferior vena cava through the nick. Cannula is now firmly tied to vena cava with the help of thread. Cannula is also fastened to the board.

   (d) A small nick is made in aorta after separating it from underlying auricle.

   (e) Frog board is fixed on the plain stand. The height of the perfusion bulb is adjusted in such a way to keep the effective venous pressure at 2-4 cm of water. Perfusion rate is kept at 40 drops per minute (counted from the bubbles in the perfusion bulb).

   (f) The thread attached to the hook through the apex of the heart is tied with lever and the tension and magnifications are adjusted. The contractions of the heart are recorded on the paper pasted on the drum of kymograph.

3. Normal tracing is taken first. Now 0.1 ml Adrenaline (1:100,000) solution is injected into the rubber tubing near the venous cannula by a tuberculin syringe. Again the tracing is obtained.

Observations:

A. Kymograph Tracing

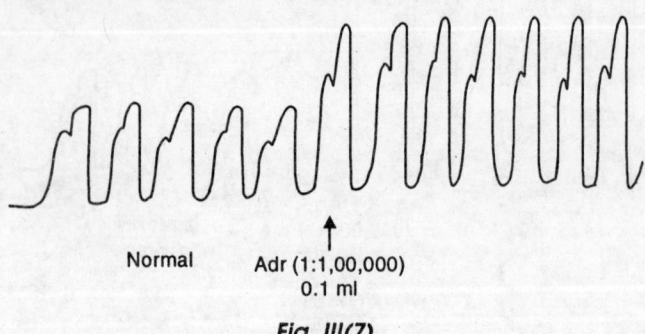

Normal   Adr (1:1,00,000)
0.1 ml

Fig. III(7)

B. Kymograph tracing shows that on addition of adrenaline, there is immediate increase in heart rate, amplitude of contraction and tone. The action of adrenaline is short lasting.

Inference:

Adrenaline produces the stimulation of the heart i.e. increase force of contraction, tone and rate.

Viva Questions:

Q. 1. Is it an intact heart preparation or isolated heart preparation.

Ans. As the heart is not completely isolated, it is an intact heart preparation.

Q. 2. To which group of drugs adrenaline belong?

Ans. Adrenaline is a sympathomimetic drug.

Q. 3. On which receptors does adrenaline act?

Ans. Adrenaline is agonistic at both α and β adrenergic receptors.

Q. 4. Which type of adrenergic receptors are present in the heart?

Ans. Mainly β_1 adrenergic receptors are present in the heart.

Q. 5. What are the cardiac uses of adrenaline?

Ans. 1. Cardiac arrest $\rightarrow$ to stimulate heart.
2. Stokes adam's syndrome.

Q. 6. Name other cardiac stimulant drugs.

Ans. A. Sympathomimetics eg. Adrenaline, Isoprenaline, Noradrenaline
B. Parasympatholytics eg. Atropine.
C. Directly acting stimulants eg. calcium chloride ($CaCl_2$)

Q. 7. How will you test that the given drug is sympathomimetic and not directly acting?

Ans. Propanolol (β-Blocker) is given in the rubber tubing and then drug is added. If the stimulant action of the drug is not present now, it means it is blocked by β-Blocker. So, the drug is acting via β-receptors. therefore it is sympathomimetic.

EXPERIMENT NO. 2

Aim:

To study the effect of acetylcholine on perfused frog's heart in situ.

Requirements:

Same as in Experiment No. 1 except acetylcholine (1:100,000) is required in place of adrenaline.

Procedure:

The experiment is performed in the same way as Experiment No. 1 except that 0.1 ml of acetylcholine (1:100,000) is added to the rubber tubing in place of adrenaline.

Observations:

A. Kymograph Tracing

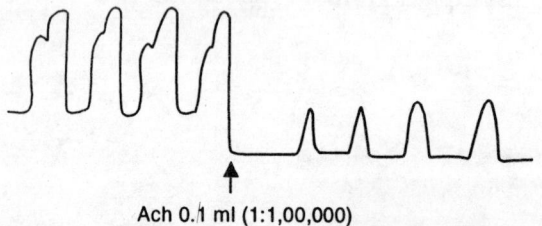

Ach 0.1 ml (1:1,00,000)

Fig. III(8)

B. From the Kymograph tracing it is seen that on adding acetylcholine there is
   - decrease in tone as indicated by downward shift in baseline
   - decrease in amplitude
   - decrease in heart rate

Inference:

Acetylcholine decreases the heart rate, tone and amplitude of heart thereby acts as depressant of heart.

Viva Questions

Q. 1. To which group of drugs do acetylcholine belongs?

Ans. Acetylcholine is a parasympathomimetic drug.

Q. 2. On which type of receptors do it act?

Ans. Acetylcholine acts by stimulating nicotinic and muscarinic cholinergic receptors.

Q. 3. Which type of cholinergic receptors are present in heart?

Ans. M_2 muscarinic receptors.

Q. 4. Can the action of acetylcholine on heart be blocked by atropine?

Ans. Yes, atropine blocks the action of acetylcholine on heart.

Q. 5. Why do atropine is used as blocker of Acetylcholine in frog's perfused heart experiment whereas d-tubocurarine is used as blocker of acetylcholine in case of frog rectus abdominis muscle preparation?

Ans. Because in the heart, ACh produces its effects by acting on muscarinic (M_2) receptors and in the rectus muscle, it acts at neuromuscular junction by acting on Nicotinic (N_M) receptors. As atropine is a blocker of muscarinic receptors and d-Tuboucrarine is a blocker of nicotinic receptors, therefore Atropine is used in heart experiments and dTC is used in muscle experiments.

Q. 6. Name other cardiac depressant drugs?

Ans. 1. Parasympathomimetics - ACh
     2. Sympatholytics - Propanolol (β-Blocker)
     3. Directly Acting - Potassium chloride (KCl)

Q. 7. Why acetylcholine is not used clinically?

Ans. Acetylcholine is not used clinically because
   1. It is rapidly hydrolysed by plasma cholinesterase according to the reaction.

$$ACh \xrightarrow{\text{cholinesterase}} Acetate + Choline$$

Due to the degradation reaction, ACh is not available to act and so, is not used therapeutically.

   2. It has very non-specific action. It acts on all types of nicotinic and cholinergic receptors, thus producing severe side effects.

Q. 8. How will you test that the given drug is parasympathomimetic and not directly acting depressant?

Ans. Atropine is given in the rubber tubing and then the drug is added. If the depressant action of the drug disappears, that means it is blocked by atropine, so it is a parasympathomimetic drug. If the action is not blocked, then it is directly acting.

EXPERIMENT NO. 3

Aim:

To study the effect of atropine on perfused frog's heart in situ.

Requirement:

Same as in Experiment No. 1 and also 1:100,000 ACh solution and 1:10,000 atropine sulphate solution.

Procedure:

1. Set up and mounting of heart is done as in Experiment No. 1 & Baseline graph is taken.

2. 0.1 ml of 1:100,000 Adrenaline is injected into the rubber tubing and tracing is taken.

3. After washing, baseline is again recorded and now 0.1 ml 1:100,000 ACh is added. The graph is again taken. (Adrenaline and acetylcholine are added to check the sensitivity/responsiveness of tissue).

4. After washing again graph is taken and baseline recorded. Now 0.1 ml atropine sulphate (1:10,000) is added to the rubber tubing and effect is recorded.

5. Without washing, ACh 0.1 ml is added to the rubber tubing, to know that whether effect of ACh is blocked or not.

Observations:

A. Kymograph Tracing

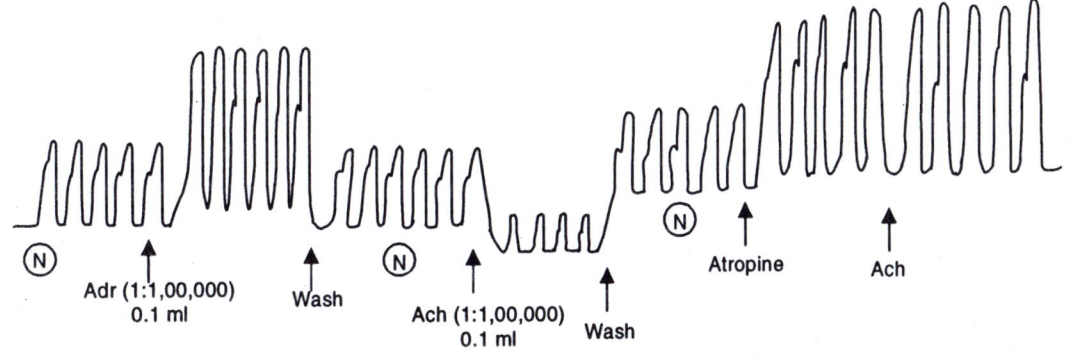

Fig. III(9)

B. From the Kymograph tracing it is noted that.
   - Tissue is sensitive to drugs as manifested by stimulation of heart on addition of Adr & depression of heart by Ach.
   - On adding atropine, there is increase in heart rate, tone and amplitude of contractions. But this increase is less as compared to adrenaline.
   - On adding ACh again, there is no depression of heart i.e. the effect of ACh is blocked.

Inference:

Atropine acts as a stimulant of heart by blocking the action of Ach. So, it is a parasympatholytic drug.

Viva Questions

Q. 1. What is the source of atropine?

Ans. It is obtained from plant *Atropa belladona*.

Q. 2. To which group of drugs do atropine belong?

Ans. Atropine is an anticholinergic or parasympatholytic drug.

Q. 3. What are the clinical indications of atropine?

Ans. It is used as

1. Antisecretory agent in pre anaesthetic medication.
2. Pain reliever in intestinal and renal colic.
3. Mydriatic for refraction testing in children.
4. Cardiac vagolytic in digitalis toxicity.

5. Antidote for early mushroom poisoning and anticholinesterase poisoning (organophosphate and carbamate poisoning).

Q. 4. What is the main contraindication of atropine?

Ans. It is contraindicated in glaucoma patients.

Q. 5. Which chemical substance is responsible for Dhatura poisoning?

Ans. Atropine

Q. 6. What is the difference in action of atropine and adrenaline (or calcium chloride) on heart?

Ans. 1. Atropine produces less marked stimulation of heart than $CaCl_2$ or adrenaline.

2. Effect of Adrenaline and $CaCl_2$ is short lasting whereas in case of atropine, the effect is long lasting.

Q. 7. Name various types of cholinergic receptors and the sites where these are present?

Ans. There are two types of cholinergic receptors

(1) *Muscarinic Receptors* – *Site*

M_1 – Autonomic ganglia
Gastric Glands
CNS

M_2 – Heart

M_3 – Smooth Muscle
Glands

(2) Nicotinic Receptors

N_M – Neuromuscular junction

N_N – Autonomic ganglia
Adrenal medulla
CNS

EXPERIMENT NO. 4

Aim:

To study the effect of calcium chloride on perfused frog's heart in situ.

Requirements:

Same as in Experiment No. 1 and also ACh (1:100,000) solutions, calcium chloride (1%).

Procedure:

1. Set up and mounting of the heart is done as in Experiment No. 1.
2. Sensitivity of the heart to ACh and Adr is checked as in Experiment No. 3.
3. After baseline recording, 0.1 ml of $CaCl_2$ is added in the rubber tubing.
4. Tracing is taken and then after washing Propanlol (β-Blocker) is added and without washing $CaCl_2$ is again added. The tracing is recorded to know whether effect of stimulant drug is blocked or not.

Observations:

(1) Kymograph Tracing [Fig. III(10)]
(2) From the tracing it is observed that
   - Tissue is sensitive to Adr and Ach.
   - $CaCl_2$ stimulates the heart as it increases the heart rate, force of contraction and tone.
   - Effect of the stimulant drug is not blocked by β-Blocker

Inference:

$CaCl_2$ increases the force of contraction and tone

which is not blocked by propanolol (β-Blocker). Thus, it is directly acting stimulant.

Viva Questions

Q. 1. What is the difference in the action of $CaCl_2$ from that of adrenaline on frog's heart?

Ans. There was little change is heart rate with $CaCl_2$ whereas with Adrenaline there is marked increase in heart rate. Tone and amplitude increases with Both. Onset of action with $CaCl_2$ is slower but more sustained as compared to Adr. On giving high doses of $CaCl_2$ heart stops in systole.

Q. 2. How will you confirm that the given drug is $CaCl_2$?

Ans. On increasing the dose of $CaCl_2$, tone increases markedly and the heart stops in systole.

Q. 3. What are the clinical uses of calcium?

Ans. 1. Immediate treatment of tetany (Calcium gluconate)
   2. As dietary supplement in growing children, pregnant, lactating and menopausal women.
   3. As an adjuvant to Hormone Replacement Therapy.
   4. Treatment of Hyperkalemia (calcium gluconate).

Q. 4. How do the mechanism of action of Adrenaline and $CaCl_2$ differ?

Ans. Adrenaline acts via $β_1$ receptor to produce stimulation of heart whereas $CaCl_2$ acts directly.

Q. 5. What are the normal serum levels of calcium?

Ans. 8.5 - 11.0 mEq/L.

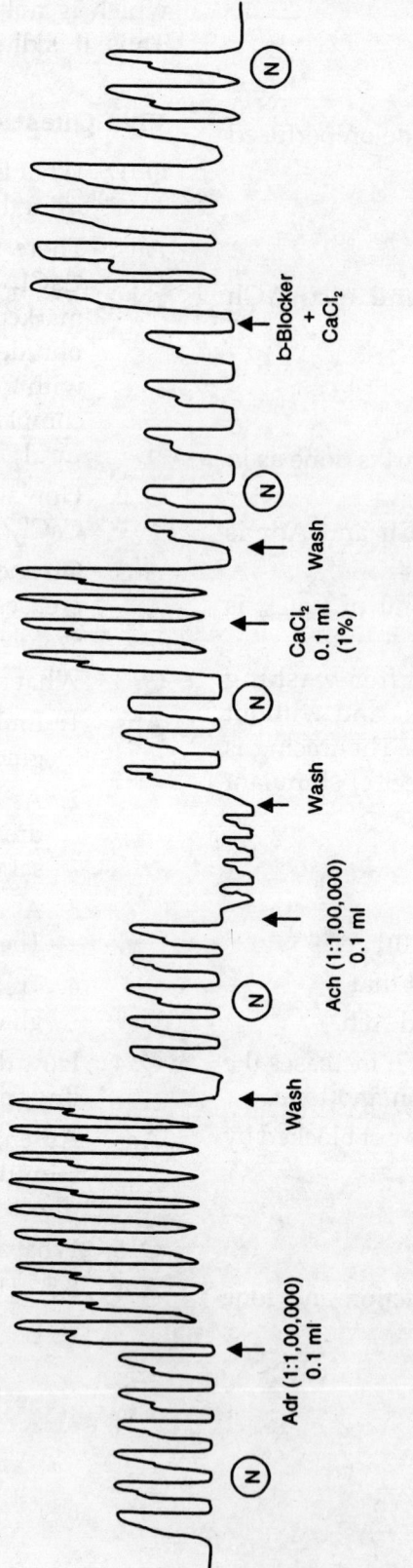

Fig. III(10)

EXPERIMENT NO. 5

Aim:

To study the effect of potassium chloride on perfused frog's heart in situ.

Requirements:

As in Experiment No. 1 and also 1:100,000 acetylcholine solution and 1% potassium chloride solution.

Procedure:

1. Set up and mounting of heart is done as in Experiment No. 1 and base line graph is taken.
2. Sensitivity of tissue is tested for acetylcholine and adrenaline as in Experiment No. 3.
3. After recording baseline contraction, 0.1 ml of 1% KCl solution is added to the rubber tubing and tracing is obtained.
4. After washing, 0.1 ml of atropine is added and after that 0.1 ml of KCl is added again and the tracing is obtained. This step is done to know whether the effect of depressant drug is blocked by atropine or not.

Observations:

A. Kymograph Tracing [Fig. III(11)]
B. From the Kymograph tracing it is observed that
   – tissue is sensitive to adrenaline and acetylcholine.
   – On adding KCl, depressant effect on heart is seen manifested by decrease in heart rate, amplitude and tone of contractions
   – The depressant action of KCl is not blocked by atropine

Inference:

Potassium chloride is a depressant drug for heart and as its effect is not blocked by atropine, it is directly acting depressant.

Viva-Questions

Q. 1. How will you confirm that the given drug is KCl?
Ans. When the depressant effect of the drug is not blocked by atropine, it is likely to be directly acting depressant like KCl. For confirming it, a large dose of the drug is given which results in stopping the heart in diastole.
Q. 2. What is the normal serum levels of potassium?
Ans. 2.5 – 5.0 mEq/L.
Q. 3. How do the mechanism of action of acetylcholine and KCl differ?
Ans. ACh acts on the heart via M_2 receptors whereas KCl acts directly.
Q. 4. What other group of the drugs may be responsible for myocardial depression?
Ans. β-Blockers like propanolol.

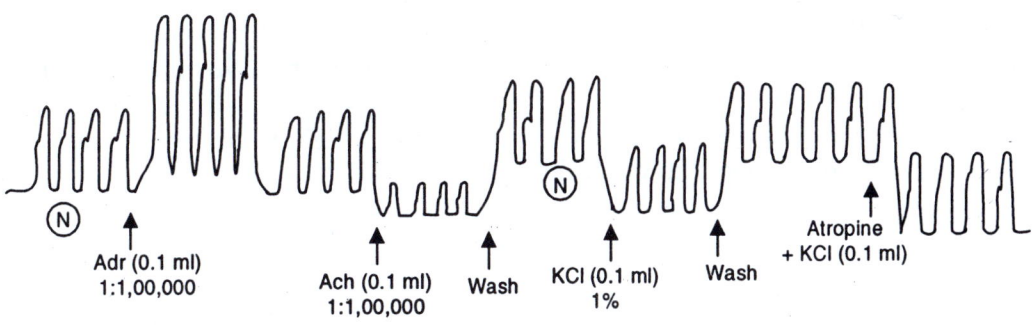

Fig. III(11)

EXPERIMENT NO. 6

Aim:

To identify the nature of unknown drug by its action on perfused frog's heart in situ.

Requirements:

Kymograph, frog board, dissection set, perfusion apparatus (perfusion bulb fitted with cork and glass tube, rubber tubing, venous cannula, retort stand with a ring for holding the perfusion bulb), iron stand, frontal writing lever, thread, pins, tuberculin syringe, pithing needle, frog's ringer solution, adrenaline (1:100,000), acetylcholine (1:100,000), unknown drug and a large or medium sized frog.

Procedure:

(1) Setting of the apparatus and mounting of the heart is done as is Experiment No. 1.

(2) Sensitivity of the heart to adrenaline and acetylcholine is checked as in Experiment No. 3.

(3) After obtaining base line tracing, 0.1 ml of unknown drug is injected in the rubber tubing and graph is recorded. The experiment is proceeded further by noticing whether the unknown drug is stimulant or depressant of heart.

If the Unknown Drug is Stimulant of Heart

If the unknown drug is stimulant of heart, the possibilities are

• Parasympatholytic (Atropine)

• Sympathomimetic (Adrenaline)

• Directly acting stimulant ($CaCl_2$)

If the drug is stimulant, the experiment is proceeded as follows:

(a) Without washing the unknown drug, acetylcholine is added to the rubber tubing. If the depressant action of acetylcholine is blocked by the unknown drug, then it must be atropine and if there is depression of heart after adding Ach, then step (b) is performed.

(b) After washing, 0.1 ml of 1:10,000 propranolol (β-Blocker) is added. Now one minute is given for propanolol to block all the receptors and without washing unknown drug is added. If the stimulant action of the unknown drug is blocked, then it is sympathomimetic like adrenaline and if the effect is not blocked (i.e. unknown drug still produces stimulation); then it must be directly acting stimulant like $CaCl_2$. Sympathomimetic drugs (like adrenaline) can be confirmed by direct matching.

If the Unknown Drug is Depressant of Heart

If the unknown drug causes depression of heart, there are again three possibilities.

– Parasympathomimetic (Acetylcholine)

– Sympatholytic (β-Blockers like propanolol)

– Directly acting depressant like KCl.

Propanolol is not given as unknown drug in the examination. So, the unknown depressant can be either parasympathomimetic or sympatholytic. To know the nature of unknown depressant, the experiment is proceeded as follows:

After washing 0.1 ml of atropine (1:10,000) is added and after waiting for one minute, unknown drug is again added. If the depressant action of unknown drug disappears, it must be parasympathomimetic like acetylcholine and if depressant action is still present, it should be directly acting drug like KCl. To confirm Ach, direct matching is done and to confirm KCl, large dose of unknown drug is added, if the heart stops in diastole, it confirms KCl.

Flow-Chart to determine nature of Unknown Drug

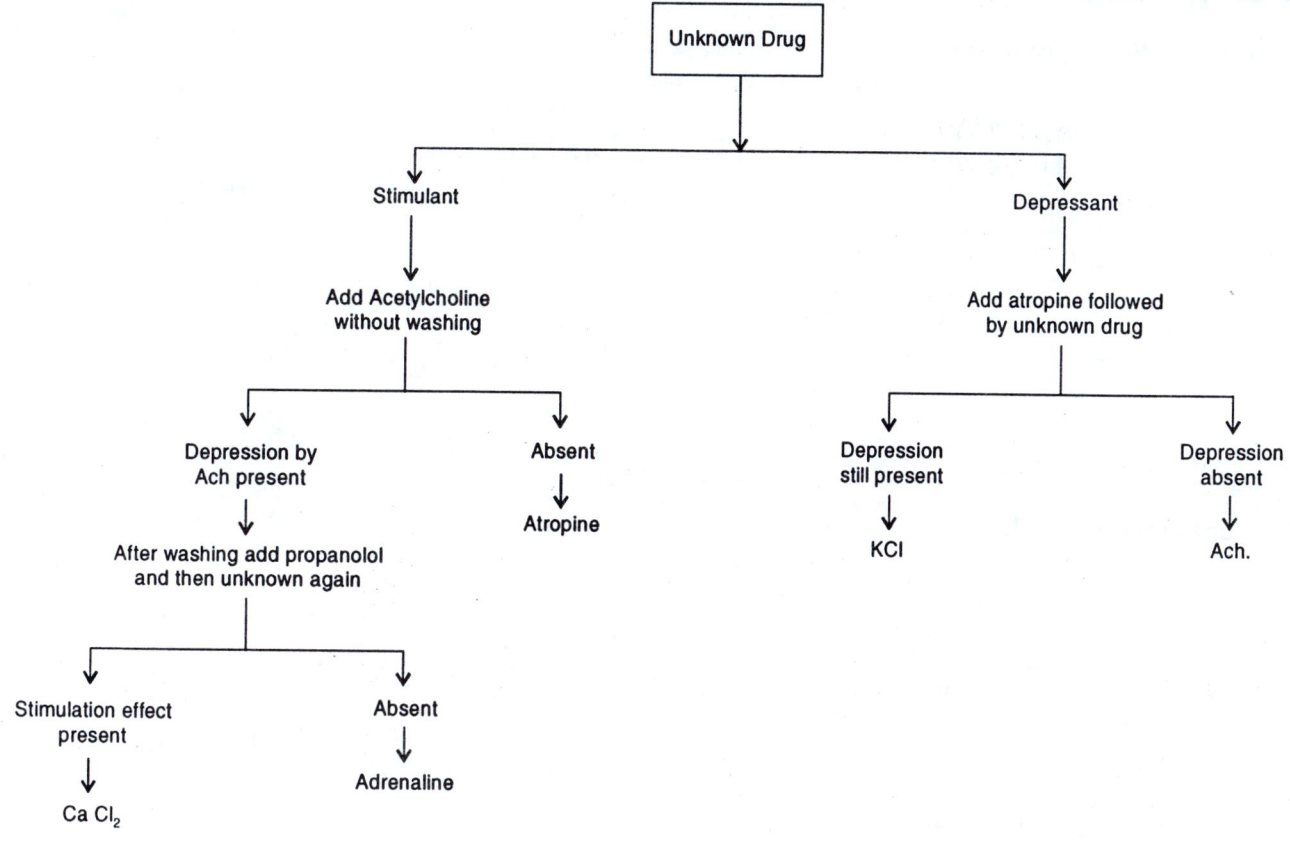

Observations:

Kymograph tracings are pasted in the practical file.

1. If unknown is adrenaline

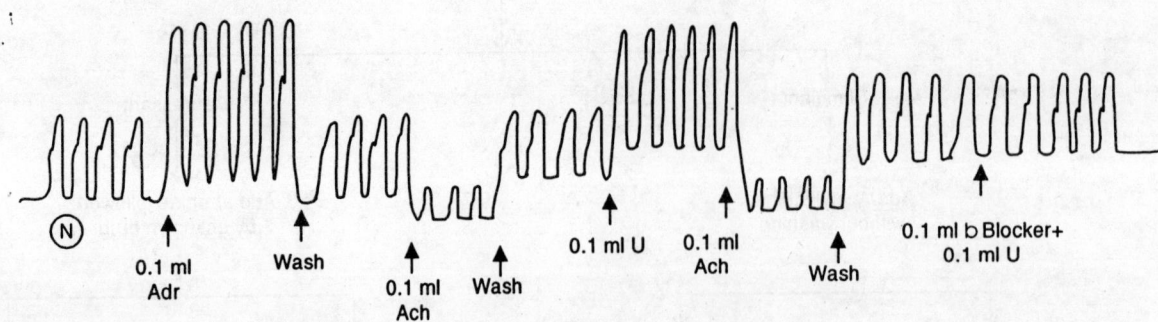

Fig. III(12)

2. If unknown is CaCl$_2$

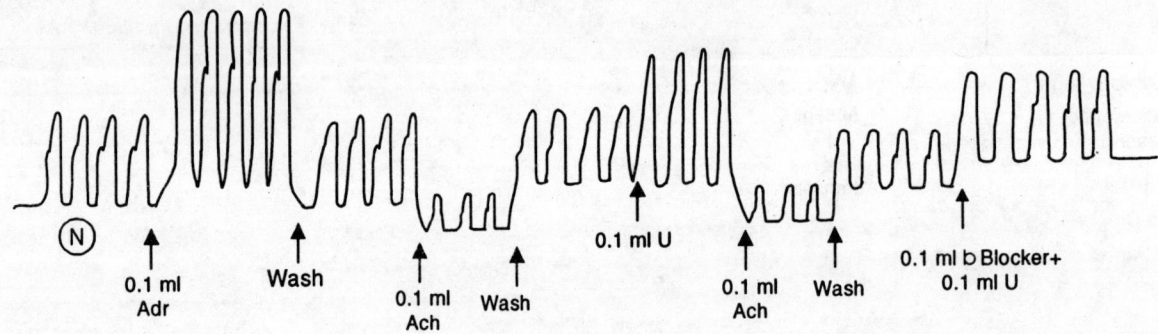

Fig. III(13)

3. If unknown is atropine

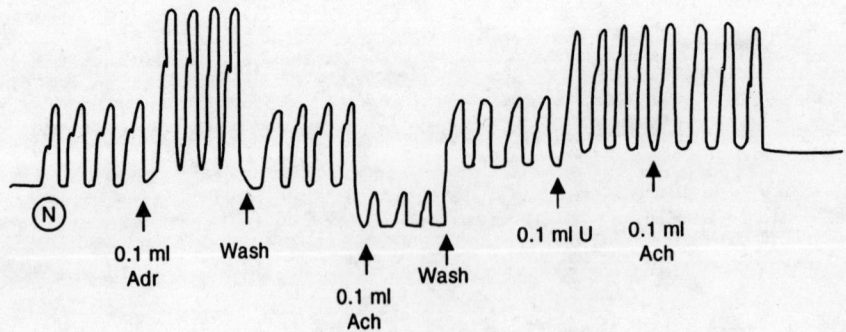

Fig. III(14)

4. If the unknown is Ach

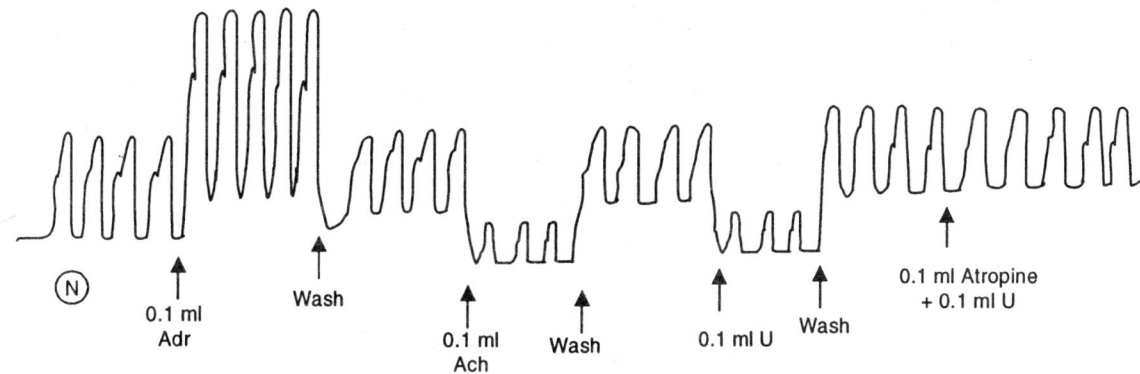

Fig. III(15)

5. If the unknown is KCl

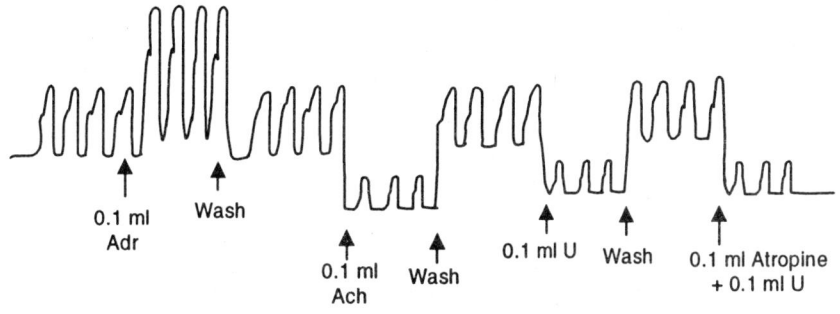

Fig. III(16)

Viva Questions

Q. 1. Which type of preparation is this, intact or isolated?

Ans. Intact perfused frog's heart in situ.

Q. 2. What is the difference between intact and isolated heart experiments?

Ans. In case of isolated heart experiments, only the direct effects of the drugs on heart will be manifested whereas in case of intact heart preparations, both direct as well as reflex effects are produced. Immediate effects are due to direct effect and after some time reflex effects appear.

Q. 3. What is the effective venous pressure in your preparation?

Ans. 2-4 cm of water.

Q. 4. From where do the frog heart gets its oxygen supply?

Ans. Oxygen is obtained from that dissolved in perfusion fluid (Frog Ringer). Extra oxygen is not required as it is sufficient.

Q. 5. What are cardiotonic drugs? How do they differ from cardiac stimulants?

Ans. Cardiotonic drugs are those drugs which result in increase in tone of heart contractions i.e. force of contraction increases. Heart rate may be increased or decreased. On the other hand, cardiac stimulants increase the heart rate, tone and amplitude. Digoxin is an example of cardiotonic drug which increases force of contraction whereas decrease heart rate.

Q. 6. What is the concentration of adrenaline and acetylcholine used?

Ans. Adrenaline and acetylcholine are used in concentration of 1:100,000. It means 1g of drug is present in 100,000 ml of solution which is equivalent to 10 μg/ml.

Q. 7. What are the main precautions to be kept in mind in this experiment?

Ans. 1. Heart tissue should not be pinched with forceps.
2. Prevent the heart from drying by application of frog ringer solution at regular intervals.
3. Ventricle should not be punctured while passing the pin through its apex.

Q. 8. What are the concentrations of Blockers (Atropine and propanolol) used in this experiment?

Ans. 1:10,000 means 100 μg/ml.

Q. 9. After adding the blockers (atropine or propanolol), the unknown drug is added after waiting for atleast one minute. Why?

Ans. This time is given for the blockers to block all the receptors so that the unknown drug, (if sympathomimetic or parasympathomimetic) donot show its effect in presence of blockers.

Q. 10. How will you differentiate between directly acting stimulant and sympathomimetic agent?

Ans. Stimulant effect of a sympathomimetic agent is blocked by propanolol whereas it is not blocked if the unknown agent is directly acting.

Q. 11. How will you differentiate between directly acting depressant and parasympathomimetic agent?

Ans. On addition of atropine, the depressant effect of parasympathomimetic agent disapears whereas in case of directly acting drug, it persists.

Q. 12. What happens if very high dose of $CaCl_2$ or KCl is given?

Ans. In case of both the drugs, the heart stops. On giving very high dose of $CaCl_2$ the heart stops is systole whereas in case of KCl, heart stops in diastole.

Q. 13. What are the cardiovascular uses of adrenaline?

Ans. 1. To stimulate heart in cardiac arrest
2. Stokes adam's syndrome

Q. 14. What are the cardiac uses of digoxin?

Ans. 1. Congestive Heart Failure
2. Atrial Fibrillation and Flutter (To control ventricular rate)
3. Paroxysomal Supra ventricular Tachycardia (PSVT)

Q. 15. What are cardiovascular uses of propanolol?

Ans. β-Blockers are used in

1. Hypertension
2. Angina pectoris
3. Cardiac arrythmias
4. Myocardial Infarction
5. Congestive Heart Failure
6. Hypertrophic cardiomyopathy
7. Dissecting Aortic Aneurysm.

Q. 16. What are the therapeutic uses of atropine in relation to cardiovascular system?

Ans. It is used as cardiac vagolytic in digitalis toxicity.

NOTES

_____

_____

_____

_____

_____

_____

NOTES

NOTES

3. FROG RECTUS

GENERAL

Apparatus

1. *Kymograph*: It is used for obtaining the graph. The details has been described in rabbit ileum experiment.

2. *Isolated Organ Bath*: Dale's organ bath used in rabbit ileum experiment can be used here. There is no need to fill the water in the outer bath.

3. *Simple writing lever* {Fig. III(17)}: It is simplest of the levers. One end is connected to the frog rectus with the help of a thread and other end is connected with ink writing recorder.

4. *Air Bubbler and Aeration Tube:* Described in rabbit ileum experiment.

Theory:

Frog's rectus abdominis muscle is a skeletal muscle. The drugs causing muscle contraction acts on the nicotinic receptors present at the neuro-muscular junction. Normally the contraction is mediated via acetylcholine which acts on nicotinic receptors. In the examination, unknown drug will be given and its effect has to be found whether it potentiates or blocks the action of Ach. The drugs used will be

1. Physostigmine – acetylcholine esterase inhibitor

2. d-Tubocurarine – neuromuscular blocker.

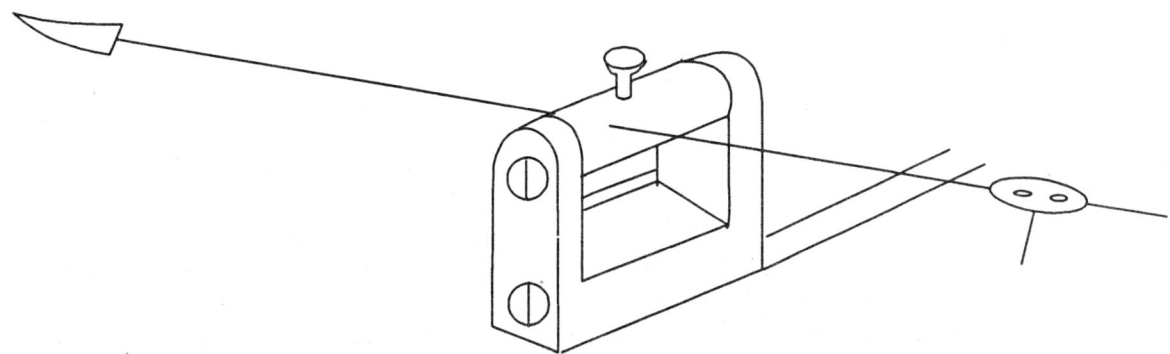

Fig. III(17) *Simple Writing Lever*

EXPERIMENT NO. 1

Aim:

(a) To demonstrate the stimulant action of acetylcholine on the frog's rectus abdominis muscle.

(b) To see the effect of increasing dosage of Acetylcholine

(c) To plot the dose response curve

(d) To plot the log dose response curve.

Apparatus Required:

Kymograph, isolated organ bath, simple writing lever, ink writing recorder, air bubbler connected with aeration tube, syringe, frog's ringer solution, acetycholine chloride solution (1:10,000), frog, scale, graph paper, dissection set.

Procedure:

1. *Adjustment of Kymograph:* Kymograph paper of suitable size is fixed on the drum and the speed of the drum is adjusted to minimum value of 0.25 mm/sec.

2. *Adjustment of Lever:* (a) The lever used in this experiment is simple writing lever. It belongs to type I lever i.e. the fulcrum or pivot lies between the writing point and point of attachment of the tissue.

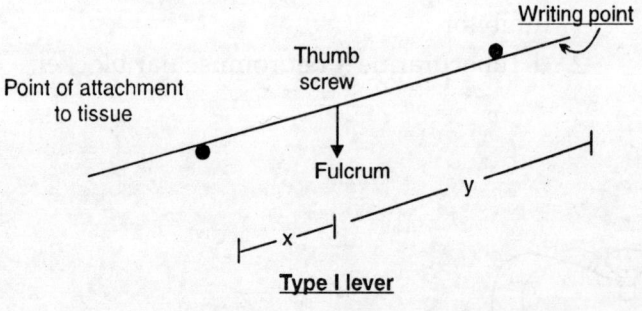

Type I lever

Fig. III(18)

The magnification of the actual contractions is adjusted by using the thumb screw, where the lever is fixed. Ink marker is attached to the end of long arm and muscle is attached to the end of short arm. Magnification is given by ratio of length of long arm to length of short arm. From the figure,

$$\text{Magnification} = \frac{y}{x}$$

The magnification of 5 is kept by adjusting the relative distances between long arm and short arm.

(c) The lever is balanced by adding plasticene on the short arm, near its end.

3. *Dissection of Frog:* A moderate sized frog is chosen, it is pithed and fixed on the frog board by laying it on its back. The skin covering the abdomen is nicked first and then cut away. Two recti are exposed. These extend from pelvic girdle to its insertion in the pectoral girdle. An incision is given over the white line in the middle, which divides it into two parts. Two threads are tied near the origin and insertion respectively. Now the muscle is cut. One end of the muscle is attached to aeration tube and inserted in the inner bath and the other end is tied to the shorted limb of lever.

4. Inner bath is filled with frog's ringer solution. The oxygenation of the fluid is done by air bubbler through the aeration tube. The muscle is now allowed to relax for 30 minutes by putting 5 gm weight on the longer limb of lever so that the fibres of muscle are stretched. Care is taken so that the muscle and thread do not touch any part of the equipment. The ringer solution is changed after every 10 minutes. After 30 minutes, the extra weight of 5 gm is removed, and the lever is adjusted so that it can touch the drum tangentially. Ringer is again changed in the inner bath. Drum is now switched on at the speed of 0.25 mm/s and the base line is drawn for 30s. Since the frog is a cold blooded animal maintenance of temperature at 37° C is not required.

5. 0.1 ml of acetylcholine (1:10,000 dilution) is added to inner bath and recordings are taken for 90s. The drum is now switched off. Ringer is changed and filled upto same level. Now, the muscle is allowed to relax for 5 minutes by hanging 5 gm weight on longer arm. Washing of the ringer is repeated. The extra weight of 5 gram is now removed and double the amount of acetylcholine (0.2 ml) is now added. Graph is again recorded for 90s and the same cycle is repeated. In this way, the recording is continued by doubling the concentration each time, till a supramaximal response is obtained. (Supramaximal response is the dose after which there is no increase in response even after

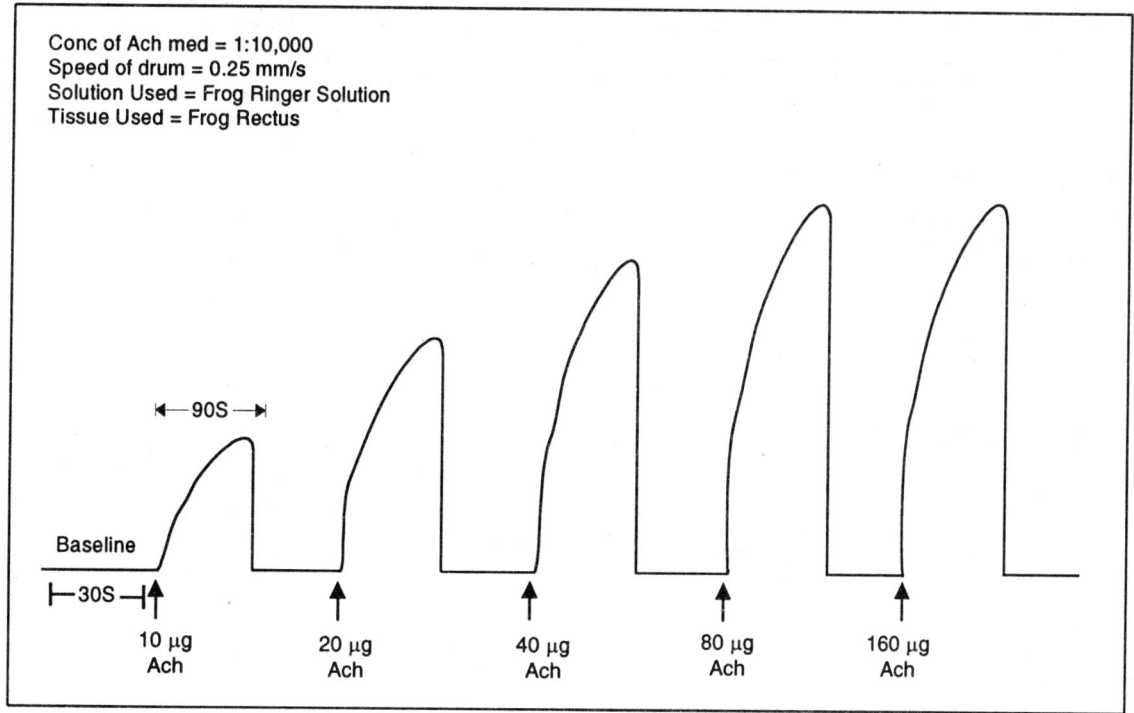

Fig. III(19)

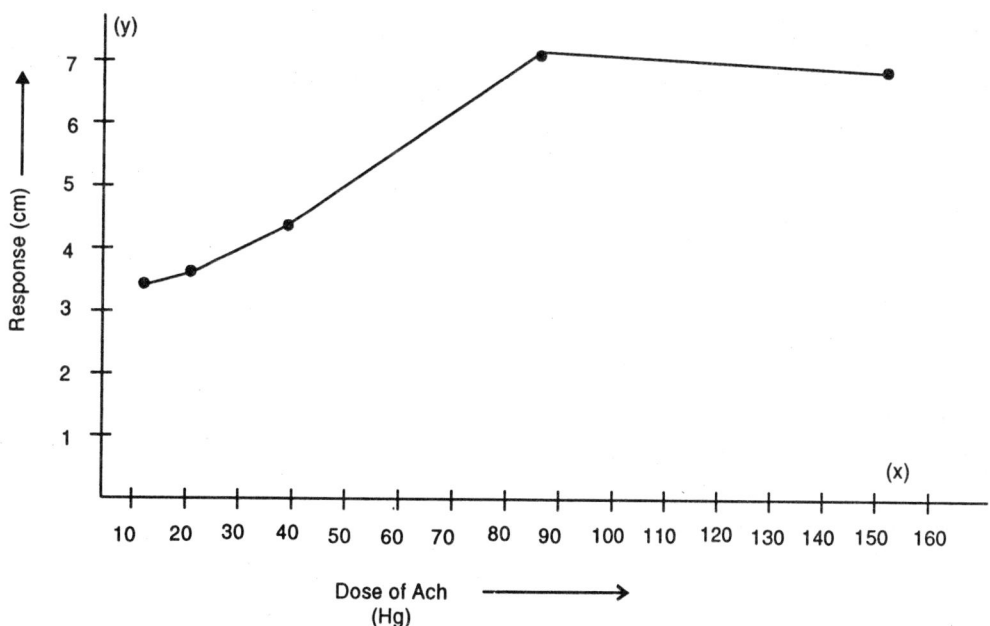

Fig. III(20)

increasing the dose). The reaching of this steady state is known as ceiling effect and the dose at which ceiling effect is achieved is called ceiling dose.

6. *Calculations:* The concentration of the drug is calculated as:

1:10,000 acetylcholine means.

10,000 ml of distilled water contains 1 gm Ach

$\therefore$ 10,000 ml of distilled water contains 1000 mg Ach

$\therefore$ 1 ml of distilled water contains $\dfrac{1000}{10,000}$ mg Ach

$\therefore$ 0.1 ml of distilled water contains

$$\dfrac{1000}{10,000} \times 0.1 \text{ mg Ach}$$

or $\dfrac{1000}{10,000} \times 0.1 \times 1000$ μg Ach

or 10 μg Ach

That means 10 μg of acetylcholine is present in 0.1 ml of the solution.

Now the concentration of the drug in the bath is calculated as.

Concentration of drug in bath =

$$\dfrac{\text{Amount of drug added}}{\text{Volume of fluid in inner bath}}$$

$$= \dfrac{10}{\pi R^2 . h} \text{ μg/ml}$$

where - R - radius of inner bath

h - height of ringer in inner bath.

Observations:

The observations are recorded as.

(1) *Recording on Kymograph Paper:* The recording of the kymograph shows that with increase in dose of acetylcholine, the muscle contraction increases and after reaching a ceiling dose there is no increase in contraction of rectus abdominis muscle

From the recording shown in Fig. III(19) it is clear that the response increase with dose of ACh till the ceiling dose of 80 μg is reached.

(2) *Dose Response Curve:* The observations are recorded as the following Table.

S.No.	Dose of ACh (μg)	Response (cm)
1.	10	3.4
2.	20	3.6
3.	40	4.7
4.	80	7.8
5.	160	7.2

A graph is now plotted with the dose on the X-axis and response on Y-axis.

From the Fig. III(20), it is found that the dose response curve is of sigmoid shape.

(3) *Log dose Response Curve:* The observations are now plotted according to table

S. No.	Dose of ACh (μg)	Log Dose	Response (in cm)
1.	10	1.000	3.4
2.	20	1.3010	3.6
3.	40	1.6021	4.7
4.	80	1.9031	7.8
5.	160	2.2041	7.2

The graph is now plotted with log dose on x-axis and response on Y-axis.

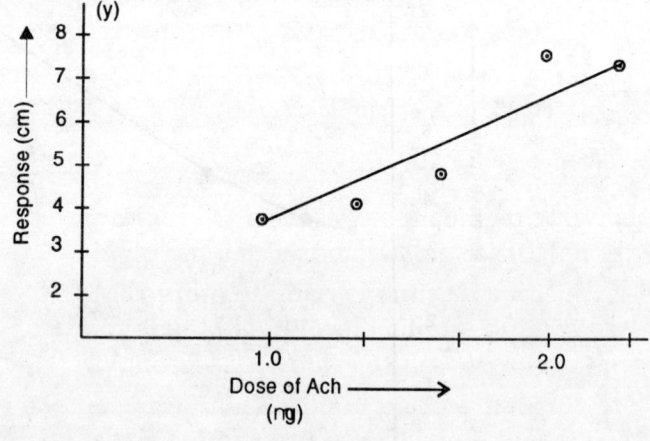

Fig. III(21)

From the Fig. III(21) it is found that the log dose response curve is a straight line.

Viva Questions

Q. 1. What is the temperature of the inner bath?

Ans. Temperature of the inner bath is kept at room temperature.

Q. 2. Why is the ringer not warmed in this experiment whereas it is warmed in rabbit ileum experiment?

Ans. Rabbit is a mammal and is a warm blooded (homeo-thermic) animal. The rabbit ileum requires temperature to be maintained at 37°C. So the ringer needs to be warmed to 37°C to use in rabbit ileum experiments. On the other hand, frog is a cold blooded (Poikilo-thermic) animal, it adjusts its temperature according to the environment, so ringer need not be warmed in this experiment.

Q. 3. What are the advantages of log dose response curve over the normal dose response curve?

Ans. Log dose response curve has following advantages over dose response curve.

(a) Large number of responses can be plotted in a smaller space.

(b) The linear part of the curve covers 25-75% of the responses and is the most sensitive dose area.

(c) When an unknown drug is administered with acetylcholine, comparison of the curve can show.

– whether the drug is agonist or antagonist. With agonist, the curve shifts to the left and with antagonists curve shifts to right.

– if the two curves are parallel, it shows that the two drugs are acting competitively and if the curves are not parallel, then they are non-competitive.

– when the two curves are parallel, the horizontal distance between the two curves gives the potency ratio of the two drugs.

4. What are the characteristics of the frog's rectus muscle preparation.

Ans. (i) It is a voluntary or skeletal muscle.

(ii) It is a slow contracting muscle. A slow contracting muscle has multiple innervation whereas fast contracting muscle has single innervation. Thus a fast contracting muscle like tibialis anterior will require a higher dose of ACh to produce contraction. This high dose can be achieved by giving ACh intra-arterially or by directly stimulating the nerve. As frog's rectus has multiple innervations, so ACh even in a smaller dose acts on multiple sites and produce a greater response.

(iii) skeletal muscle at neuromuscular junction contains only nicotinic receptors and not muscarinic receptors, so acetylcholine responses are not blocked by atropine but by d-tubocurarine.

Q. 7. What is the most sensitive muscle preparation to detect the presence of acetylcholine.

Ans. Dorsal muscle of leech.

Q. 8. What is the difference in the composition of frog's ringer and mammalian ringer solutions?

Ans. Mammalian ringer contains more sodium chloride, potassium chloride, calcium chloride, sodium bicarbonate and less glucose than frog ringer. The composition of the two ringer solutions is.

	Frog Ringer	Mammalian Ringer
Nacl	0.65 g/dl	0.9 g/dl
Kcl	0.014 g/dl	0.042 g/dl
$Cacl_2$	0.012 g/dl	0.024 g/dl
$NaHco_3$	0.020 g/dl	0.050 g/dl
NaH_2Po_4	0.001 g/dl	–
Glucose	0.2 g/dl	0.1 g/dl
Distt. water	100 ml	100 ml

Q. 9. What are nicotinic and muscarinic actions of acetylcholine?

Ans. (A) Muscarinic Actions

a. *Heart:* Decreased heart rate
Decreased force of contraction
Decreased conductivity

b. *Blood vessels:* Dilatation

c. Smooth Muscles
– In GIT: increased peristalsis
– Ureter: increased peristalsis
– Bladder: Detrussor contraction & trigone relaxation, leading to voiding of Bladder
– Bronchial Muscle: constriction

d. *Glands:* increased secretion leading to ↑ Sweating, ↑ Salivation, ↑ Lacrimation

e. *Eye:* Contraction of circular muscle of Iris → miosis

(B) Nicotinic Actions
  (a) *Skeletal Muscle:* Contraction
  (b) *Autonomic ganglia:* Stimulation of both sympathetic and parasympathetic ganglia.

Q. 10. Why is the contraction recorded for 90 seconds?

Ans. It takes time for all muscle fibres to contract and in 90s, almost all fibres contract and maximum contraction is obtained. If the muscle is allowed to contract for longer time, relaxation period has also to be extended, thus lengthening the experiment.

Q. 11. Why should the muscle fibres be relaxed before starting the experiment?

Ans. By handling the muscle, stimulus is produced and muscle contracts, so to have a proper contraction, muscle should be relaxed to the initial length before adding the drug.

EXPERIMENT NO. 2

Aim:

To study the effect of Physostigmine on the action of acetylcholine on frog's rectus abdominis muscle.

Apparatus Required:

Physostigmine sulphate (1 mg/ml), kept in air tight and light resistant containers. Rest is same as described in Experiment No. 1.

Procedure:

1. Adjustment of kymograph, adjustment of lever, dissection of frog's rectus abdominis muscle and mounting of the tissue is done as described in Experiment No. 1.
2. After the muscle is relaxed, 0.1 ml of acetylcholine (1:10,000) is added in the inner bath and concentration of acetylcholine (Ach) is determined which gives contraction of 1-2 cm height (As described in Experiment No. 1). The procedure is repeated with this concentration, in order to obtain at least two contractions of nearly same height.
3. Fresh ringer is now replaced in the inner bath and 0.2 ml of physostigmine solution is added. Muscle is kept relaxed by adding 5g weight on longer arm for 5 minutes. These 5 minutes are given for physostigmine to act on the muscle.
4. Now extraweight of 5g is removed and the calculated concentration of ACh is added to the inner bath without replacing the ringer. The contractions are now recorded for 90 s. The muscle is washed by replacing fresh ringer and relaxed as usual. The same procedure is repeated for recording two contractions with physostigmine and acetylcholine.

Calculations:

ACh concentration is calculated as in Experiment No. 1. Physostigmine concentration is calculated as follows.

1 ml distilled water contains – 1 mg physostigmine
0.2 ml distilled water contains – 0.2 mg physostigmine
or 0.2×1000 μg physostigmine

or 200 μg physostigmine

concentration of physostigmine in the inner bath is calculated as $= \dfrac{200}{\pi R^2 \cdot d}$

where R is radius of inner bath
d is height of ringer in inner bath.

Observations

The observations are recorded as

1. *Recording on kymograph paper* [Fig. III(22)]: The recording of the kymograph shows that on addition of physostigmine to fixed dose of Ach, the muscle contraction increases i.e. physo-stigmine potentiates the action of Ach, so it acts as agonist.
2. *Dose-Response Relation:* The observations are recorded as following table.

S.No.	Drug used	Dose (μg)	Response (cm)
1.	Ach	10	0.8
2.	Ach	20	1.5
3.	Ach	20	1.5
4.	Physostigmine + Ach	200 + 20	3.0
5.	Physostigmine + Ach	200 + 20	3.0

From the table it is clear that on adding physostigmine to fixed dose of Ach, the height of contraction increases.

Inference:

Physostigmine potentiates the action of acetylcholine. Therefore, it is an agonist of Ach.

Viva Questions

Q. 1. What is the source of physostigmine.

Ans. It is a natural alkaloid obtained from calabar bean (Physostigma venenosum)

Q. 2. What are the drugs which potentiates the action of ACh on skeletal muscles? What is the mechanism of action of these drugs.

Ans. Anticholinesterase drugs like physostigmine, neostigmine etc. potentiates the action of ACh on skeletal muscles. Anticholinesterases (or cholinesterase inhibitors) may be reversible or irreversible.

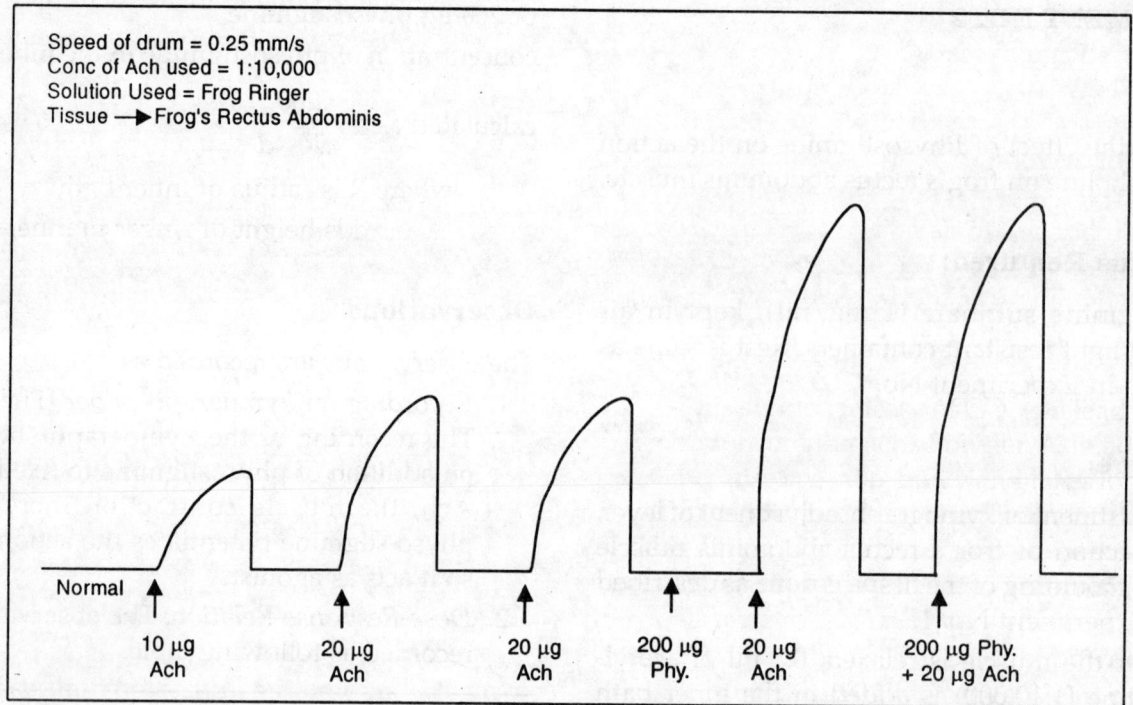

Speed of drum = 0.25 mm/s
Conc of Ach used = 1:10,000
Solution Used = Frog Ringer
Tissue → Frog's Rectus Abdominis

Normal

10 μg Ach   20 μg Ach   20 μg Ach   200 μg Phy.   20 μg Ach   200 μg Phy. + 20 μg Ach

Fig. III(22)

(a) Reversible cholinesterase inhibitors

   (i) *Carbamates* like physostigmine, neostigmine

   (ii) *Acridines* like tacrine

(b) Irreversible cholinesterase inhibitors

   (i) Organophosphates like malathion, parathion etc.

   (ii) Carbamates like carbaryl, propoxur (Baygon) etc.

Mechanism of Action: Acetylcholine is normally broken by enzyme Acetylcholinesterase into choline and acetate as

$$\text{Acetylcholine} \xrightarrow[\text{esterase}]{\text{Acetylcholine}} \text{choline} + \text{Acetate}$$

This is the main mode of termination of action of Ach.

Cholinesterase inhibitors inhibit this enzyme by either carbamylating or phosphorylating it.

Due to inhibition of this enzyme, ACh is not degraded and more of ACh is available to act on the receptors, thus potentiating its action.

Q. 3. If you draw a log dose response curve with ACh alone and Physostigmine + Ach, how will the two curves behave.

Ans. Log dose response curve of ACh alone is a straight line inclined with X-axis. The log dose response curve of Physostigmine + ACh is again a straight line parallel to the previous line. However the curve shifts towards left.

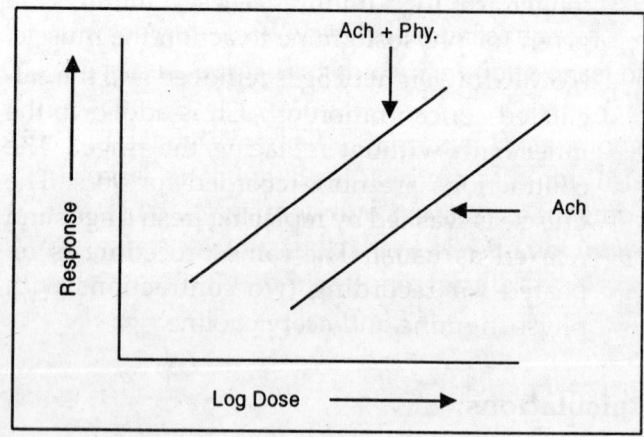

Fig. III(23)

From the Fig. III(23) it is clear that when physostigmine is added, the same response can be obtained with less concentration of ACh as obtained with ACh alone. In other words, physostigmine potentiates the action of Ach.

Q. 4. What are the therapeutic uses of Anti-cholinesterases?

Ans. Anticholinesterases are used in the following conditions.

(1) Glaucoma – as miotic, physostigmine is used.

(2) Mysthenia gravis – Neostigmine is used.

(3) Post operative paralytic ilens–Neostigmine is used

(4) Cobra Bite–Neostigmine is used.

(5) Belladona Poisoning–Physostigmine is used.

(6) Alzheimer's disease–Tacrine, Galantamine, Rivastigmine etc are used.

Q. 5. What are the drugs used in the treatment of Mystenia gravis?

Ans. 1. Neostigmine

2. Corticosteroids (Prednisolone)

3. Immunosuppresants (Azathioprine, Cyclosporine)

Q. 6. Why physostigmine is preferred over neostigmine for treatment of belladona (atropine) poisoning?

Ans. Physostigmine is a tertiary amine whereas neostigmine is a quarternary ammonium compound. Due to this structural difference physostigmine is more lipid soluble than neostigmine. Due to lipid solubility, physostigmine can cross blood brain barrier and counteract the central effects of atropine overdosage. As neostigmine cannot cross blood brain barrier, it is devoid of central effects. Therefore, physostigmine is preferred over neostigmine for treatment of belladona poisoning.

Q. 7. Why neostigmine is preferred over physostigmine for treatment of mysthenia gravis?

Ans. Mysthenia gravis is a disorder in which auto-antibodies are formed against nicotinic receptors at the muscle end plate. Neostigmine is preferred in the treatment of this disease because:

(a) Neostigmine possesses direct agonistic action on cholinoceptors whereas physostigmine is devoid of this effect.

(b) Neostigmine cannot cross blood brain barrier, therefore no central cholinergic adverse effects are present whereas physostigmine produces the central effects.

EXPERIMENT NO. 3

Aim:

To study the effect of d-Tubocurarine on the action of acetylcholine on the frog's rectus abdominis muscle.

Apparatus Required:

d-tubocurarine chloride (1 mg/ml). Rest is Same as described in Experiment No. 3.

Procedure:

1. Adjustment of kymograph, adjustment of lever, dissection of frog's rectus abdominis muscle and mounting of the tissue is done as described in Experiment No. 1.

2. After the muscle is relaxed, 0.1 ml of Acetylcholine (1:10,000) is added in the inner bath and concentration of ACh is determined which gives contraction of 1-2 cm height. The procedure is repeated with this concentration, in order to obtain at least two contractions of nearly same height.

3. Fresh ringer is now replaced in the inner bath and 0.5 ml of d-tubocurarine solution is added.

Muscle is kept relaxed by adding 5g weight on longer arm for 5 minutes.

4. Now extra weight of 5 g is removed and the calculated concentration of ACh is added to the inner bath without replacing the ringer solution. The contractions are now recorded for 90s. The muscle is washed by replacing fresh ringer and relaxed as usual. The same procedure is repeated in order to get another contraction.

Calculations:

The concentration of ACh is calculated as in Experiment No. 1.

For calculating the concentration of d-tubocurarine (dTC),
1 ml of distilled water contains – 1 mg of dTC
0.5 ml of distilled water contains – 0.5 mg of dTC
or 0.5 × 1000 µg of dTC
or 500 µg of dTC
For calculating the concentration of dTC in inner bath we use the formula; $\dfrac{500}{\pi R^2 h}$ µg/ml

Observations:

1. Recording in Kymograph Paper:

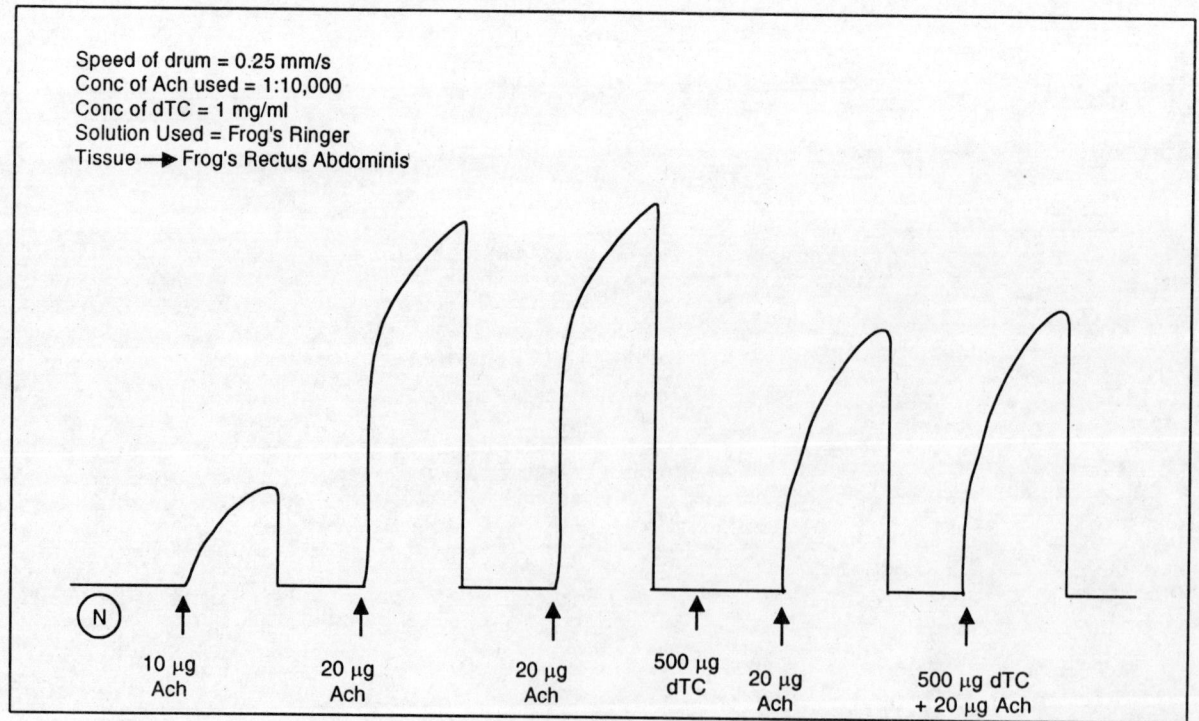

Speed of drum = 0.25 mm/s
Conc of Ach used = 1:10,000
Conc of dTC = 1 mg/ml
Solution Used = Frog's Ringer
Tissue → Frog's Rectus Abdominis

N

10 µg Ach   20 µg Ach   20 µg Ach   500 µg dTC   20 µg Ach   500 µg dTC + 20 µg Ach

Fig. III(24)

From the kymograph recordings it is clear that on giving dTC the height of contraction produced by same dose of ACh decreases. Thus dTC inhibits the action of Ach, hence the drug is an antagonist of ACh.

2. *Dose response relation:* The observations are recorded as per the following table.

S.No.	Drug	Dose (µg) (in cm)	Response
1.	Ach	10	7.0
2.	Ach	20	11.0
3.	Ach	20	11.0
4.	dTC + Ach	500 20	7.5
5.	dTC + Ach	500 20	7.5

From the table it is clear that dTC inhibits the action of ACh and thus acts as antagonist.

Inference:

d-Tubocurarine inhibits the action of Acetylcholine (ACh). Hence the drug is an antagonist of ACh.

Viva Questions

Q. 1. What is the source of d-tubocurarine?

Ans. It is obtained from strychnos toxifera, chondrodendron tomentosum and related plants.

Q. 2. What is the mechanism of action of dTC?

Ans. d-tubocurarine acts as a competetive blocker of neuromuscular junction. dTC has affinity for nicotinic (N_M) cholinergic receptors at the muscle end plate but no intrinsic activity. ACh released from motor nerve endings is not able to combine with its receptors. dTC thus reduces the frequency of channel opening. Thus it antagonises the action of ACh on skeletal muscle.

Q. 3. Which type of receptors are present in skeletal muscle?

Ans. Nicotinic cholinergic (N_M) receptors.

Q. 4. Classify skeletal muscle relaxants?

Ans. These can be classified as follows:

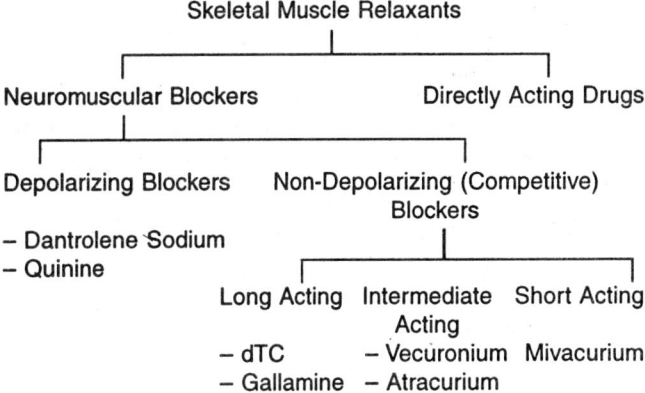

Q. 5. What is the difference in the action of d-TC and succinylcholine when added to a bath containing frog's rectus abdominis muscle?

Ans. When d-tubocurarine is added to a bath containing frog's rectus abdominis muscle, it causes inhibition of action of Ach. It acts competitively and decreases the height of contraction. On the other hand, when succinylcholine is added, it produce twitching and fasciculations first and then decreases the height of contraction. d-Tubocurarine do not produce fasciculations.

Q. 6. What are the therapeutic uses of d-tubocurarine, succinylcholine and diazepam.

Ans. 1. *d-tubocurarine:* It is not used now because of its prominent histamine releasing, ganglion blocking and cardiovascular actions as well as long duration and need for pharmacological reversal. It can be used in the provocative diagnostic test for the diagnosis of myasthenia gravis.

2. *Succinylcholine:* It is employed as an adjunct to general anaesthetics to provide good skeletal muscle relaxation. Sch is employed for brief procedures e.g. endotracheal intubation, laryngoscopy, bronchoscopy, esophagoscopy, reduction of fracture and dislocations etc. It is also used for avoiding convulsions and trauma from electroconvulsive therapy.

3. *Diazepam:* It is used as

a. sedative hypnotic

b. anxiolytic

c. anticonvulsant

d. centrally acting muscle relaxant

e. to aid in alcohol withdrawal

Q. 7. Can atropine block the action of ACh on frog's rectus abdominis muscle preparation?

Ans. No, atropine cannot block the action of ACh in this case because ACh acts on nicotinic cholinergic receptors of type N_M, to produce muscle contraction. As Atropine is a muscarinic receptor antagonist and these receptors are not involved in action of ACh on rectus abdominis muscle, atropine is not able to block the action of Ach.

Q. 8. If you draw a log dose response curve with ACh alone and ACh with d-Tubocurarine, how will the two curves behave?

Ans. The dose response curve of ACh alone is a straight line inclined at an angle to the dose axis. The dose response curve of ACh + d-Tubocurarine is also a straight line parallel to an to the right of the above mentioned line.

From the Fig. III(26) it is clear that for obtaining the same response, the concentration of ACh required is more in the presence of d-Tubocurarine. In other words, dTC inhibits the action of Ach. As the curves are parallel d-Tubocurarine acts as competitive antagonist of the Ach.

Q. 9. What are the types of antagonism?

Ans. There are two types of antagonism–competitive and non-competitive.

Competitive Antagonism (Equilibrium type)– A competitive antagonist binds to the receptor where agonist binds to produce the response. Because of occupancy of the receptor by the antagonist, agonist is not able to produce the response. In such type of antagonism, K_m is increased but V_{max} remains unchanged. If a large concentration of agonist is used, it can displace the antagonist and overcome the inhibition. Examples of the competitive antagonists are:

(a) Physostigmine and neostigmine compete with actylcholine for cholinesterase.

(b) d-Tubocurarine competes with acetylcholine for N_M receptors.

(c) Sulfonamides competes with PABA for bacterial folate synthetase.

Non-competitive Antagonism: Antagonist reacts with a site adjacent to catalytic site, but changes the enzyme in such a way that it loses its catalytic property. Therefore K_m is not changed but V_{max} decreases.

Examples of Non-competitive antagonism are

(a) Acetazolamide for carbonic anhydrase

(b) Aspirin for cyclooxygenase

(c) Disulfiram for aldehyde dehydrogenase.

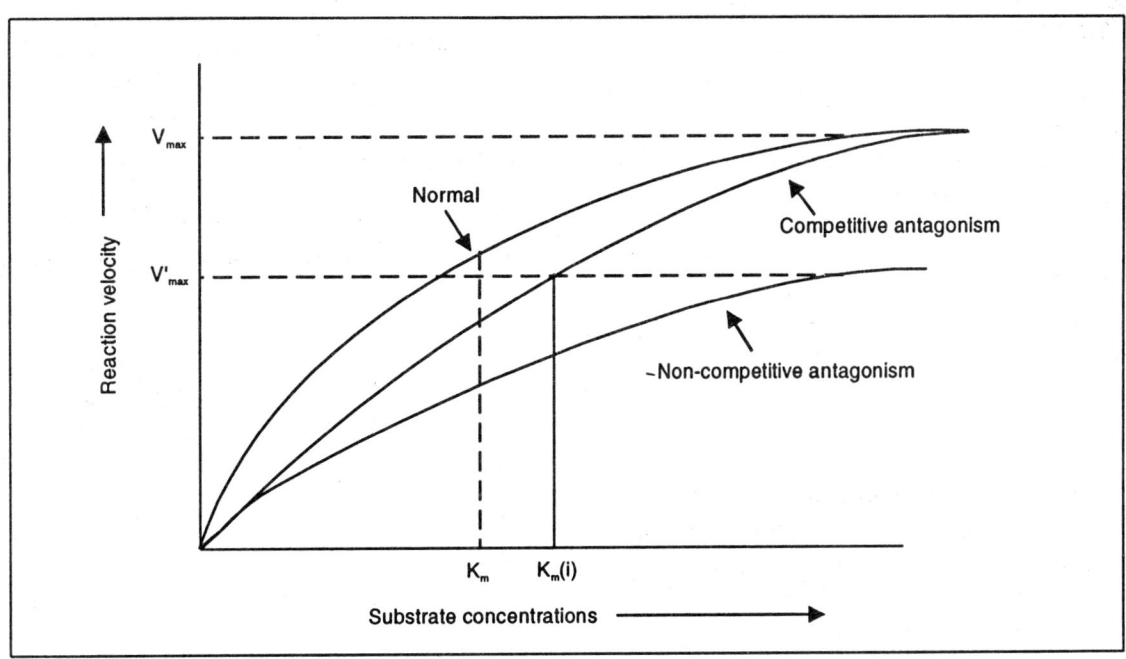

K_m – rate constant of normal reaction and of Non-competitive antagonism

K_m' – rate constant of competitive antagonism

V_{max} – Max. velocity of normal reaction and competitive antagonism

V_{max}' – Max. velocity of non-competitive antagonism

Fig. III(25)

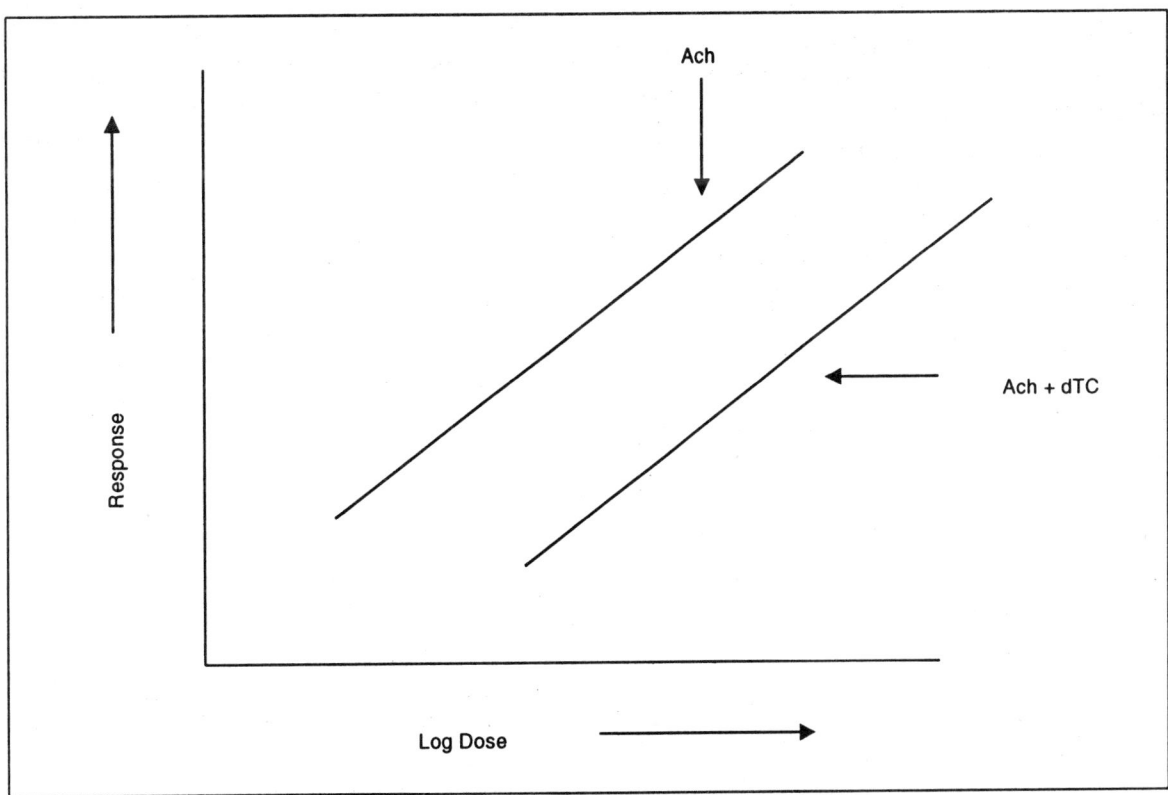

Fig. III(26)

EXPERIMENT NO. 4

Aim:

To identify the nature of unknown drug by its action on frog's rectus abdominis muscle.

Apparatus Required:

Unknown drug. The rest is same as in experiment No. 1.

Procedure:

1. Adjustment of kymograph, adjustment of lever, dissection of frog's rectus abdominis muscle and mounting of the tissue is done as described in Experiment No. 1.

2. After the muscle is relaxed, 0.1 ml of acetylcholine (1: 10,000) is added to the inner bath and that concentration of ACh is determined which gives contraction of 1-2 cm height. The procedure is repeated with this concentration, in order to obtain at least two contractions of nearly equal height.

3. Fresh ringer is now replaced in the inner bath and 0.5 ml of unknown drug solution is added. Muscle is kept relaxed by adding 5 g weight on longer arm for 5 minutes.

4. Now this extra weight is removed and the calculated concentration of ACh is added to the inner bath without replacing the ringer solution. The contractions are now recorded for 90s. The muscle is washed by replacing fresh ringer

and relaxed. The same procedure is repeated for recording two contractions.

Observations:

(1) Recording of Kymograph [Fig. III(27)]

(2) The observations are recorded in tabular form as follows.

S.No.	Drug	Dose	Height of contraction (mm)	Remarks
1.	Ach	10 µg	11	–
2.	Ach	20 µg	28	–
3.	Ach	20 µg	28	–
4.	Unknown	0.5 ml	–	No fibrillation observed
5.	U + Ach	0.5 ml + 20 µg	14	– ACh effect reduced
6.	U + Ach	0.5 ml + 20 µg	13	– ACh effect reduced

Inference:

From the observations, it is clear that the unknown drug antagonized the action of ACh on frog's rectus abdominis muscle. Also, as the drug itself donot produce fasciculations, it may be competitive blocker like d-Tubocurarine.

Viva-Questions

Same as in Experiment No. 1, 2 & 3

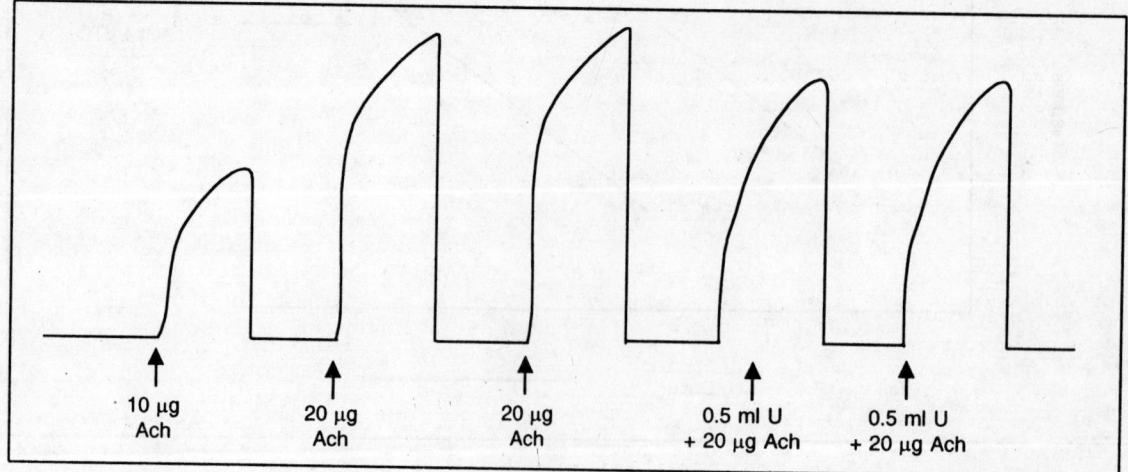

Fig. III(27)

EXPERIMENT NO. 5

Aim:

The identify the nature of unknown drug by its action on frog's rectus abdominis muscle.

Apparatus Required:

Same as in Experiment No. 4.

Procedure:

Same as in Experiment No. 4.

Observations:

1. Recording of Kymograph

2. Observations are recorded in the tabular form as follows.

S.No.	Drug	Dose	Height of contraction (mm)	Remarks
1.	Ach	10 mg	11	–
2.	Ach	20 mg	18	–
3.	Ach	20 mg	18	–
4.	Unknown	0.5 ml	–	–
5.	U + Ach	0.5 ml + 20 mg	28	U increased the effect of Ach
6.	U + Ach	0.5 ml + 20 mg	28	U increased the effect of Ach

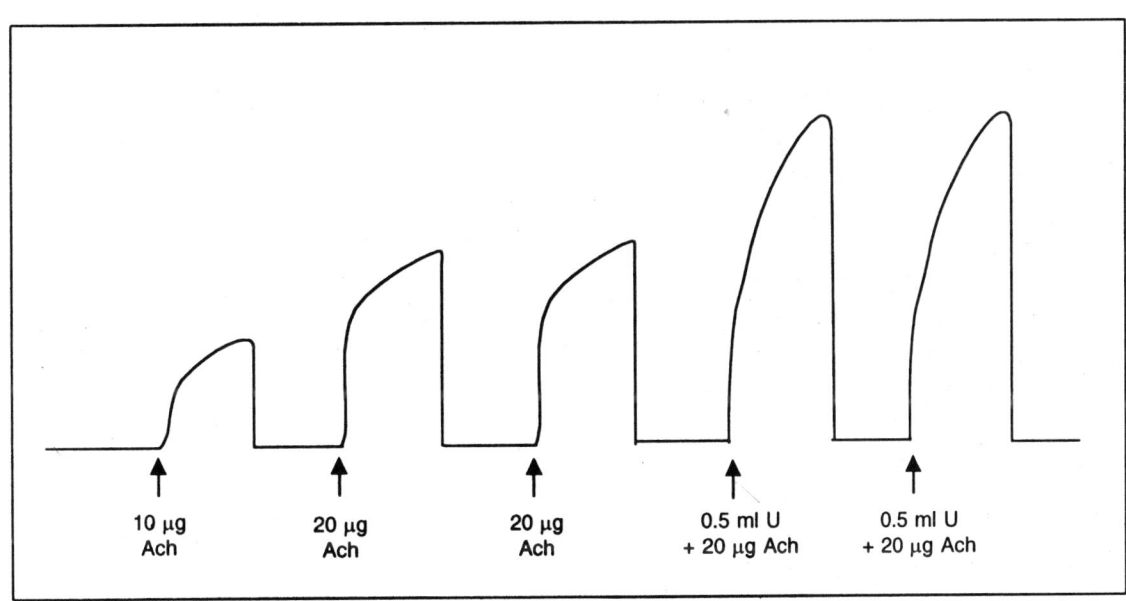

Fig. III(28)

Inference:

From the above observations, it is clear that unknown drug potentiated the action of ACh on frog's rectus abdominis muscle. So, it must be cholinesterase inhibitor like physostigmine.

Viva Questions:

Same as in Experiment 1, 2, & 3.

NOTES

NOTES

NOTES

PART-IV
PRESCRIPTION WRITING

PRESCRIPTION WRITING

GENERAL

In the examination, students are given three exercises. In one of these, student has to prescribe the drug for a particular disease state/condition. All parts of the prescription should be written properly. A *model prescription* is given here.

(1)

> Dr. Rajesh, M.D.
> 76, Basant Vihar, Delhi
> Regd. No. 2004/UCMS/642
> Dated: 9-07-2004

> Tarun Arora
> 8 year/Male
> Regd. No. 1632

(2)

> Diagnosis - Scabies

(3)

> ℞

(4a)

(4b)

Benzyl benzoate solution	.5 ml
Emulsifying wax	1.25 g
Aqua ad.	20 ml

(4c)

> Mix and make and send such 20 ml

(4d)

> Apply all over the body from neck down after a hot scrubbing bath. Repeat application after 12 hours followed by a bath with change of clothings.

> *Rajesh*
> Regd. No. 2004/UCMS/642

1. Doctor's Particulars with Date
2. Patient's Particulars
3. Diagnosis
4. (a) Superscription - Symbol ℞
   (b) Inscription   - Drugs
   (c) Subscription   - Directions to pharmacist
   (d) Signa   - Directions to patient
   (e) Initials   - Signature of the doctor along with Regd. No.

PRESCRIPTION FOR SPECIFIC MEDICAL CONDITIONS

Some important prescriptions are given in this section of the book.

1. Prescribe the drug treatment for a patient of status epilepticus.

Dr. Rajesh
76, Basent Vihar, Delhi
Regd. No. 2003/UCMS/642
Dated: 16-07-2004

Sunil
24 yr/M
Regd. No. 1213

    Δ   Status Epilepticus

Rx

    Inj. Diazepam 10 mg.

    Send such two vials.

    One vial to be injected i/v stat and other to be given if necessary.

Rajesh
2003/UCMS/642

---

*Note: Clonazepam 2 mg i/v can be used as an alternative.

2. Prescribe drug treatment for a patient of grand mal epilepsy.

Dr. Rajesh
76, Basent Vihar, Delhi
Regd. No. 2003/UCMS/642
Dated : 16-07-2004

Sunil
24 yr/M
Regd. No. 1213

    Δ   Grand Mal Epilepsy

Rx

    Tab. Carbamazepine 200 mg.

    Send such 21 tablets

    Take one tablet TDS for 7 days and review after 7 days.

Rajesh
2003/UCMS/642

---

*Note: Alternative drug is Tab. Phenytoin Sodium 100 mg TDS × 7 days and review.

3. Prescribe for a patient of petit mal epilepsy.

Dr. Rajesh
76, Basent Vihar, Delhi
Regd. No. 2003/UCMS/642
Dated: 10-07-04

Sunil
24 yr/M
Regd. No. 1213

Δ   Petit Mal Epilepsy

R

   Tab. Sodium Valproate 200 mg.

   Send such 21 tablets

   Take one tablet TDS for 7 days and review after 7 days.

Rajesh
2003/UCMS/642

Note: Ethosuximide can be used in place of sodium valproate.

4. Prescribe the drug treatment for a patient of status asthmaticus.

Dr. Rajesh
76, Basent Vihar, Delhi
Regd. No. 2003/UCMS/642
Dated: 10-07-04

Sunil
24 yr/M
Regd. No. 1213

Δ   Status Asthmaticus

R

   Inj. Hydrocortisone (100 mg) ampule

   Inj. Salbutamol (2 mg) ampule

   Inj. Ipratropium (500 μg) ampule

Send two ampules of each drug.
One ampule of hydrocortisone to be given i/v stat followed by slow intravenous infusion of another ampule of hydrocortisone in 8 hours. Nebulization with salbutamol and Ipratropium to be given intermittently and Oxygen inhalation to be given intermittently.

Rajesh
2003/UCMS/642

---

5. Prescribe the treatment for Acute Bacterial Dysentry.

Sunil
24 yr/M
Regd. No. 1213

Dr. Rajesh
76, Basent Vihar, Delhi
Regd. No. 2003/UCMS/642
Dated: 10-07-04

Δ   Acute Bacterial Dysentry

℞

Tab. Ciprofloxacin 400 mg.

Send such 10 tablets

One tablet to be taken BD per orally for 5 days.

Rajesh
2003/UCMS/642

Note: Cotrimoxazole (400 mg Sulphamethoxazole + 80 mg Trimethoprim) 2 tabs. BD × 5 days can be used as an alternative.

6. Prescribe for a patient of Helicobacter pylori infection.

Sunil
24 yr/M
Regd. No. 1213

Dr. Rajesh
76, Basent Vihar, Delhi
Regd. No. 2003/UCMS/642
Dated: 10-07-04

Δ   Helicobacter pylori infection.

℞

Tab. Lansoprazole 30 mg

Cap. Amoxycillin 1000 mg

Tab. Clarithromycin 500 mg

Send 28 tablets of each drug.

Take one tablet of each drug BD per orally for 14 days.

Rajesh
2003/UCMS/642

7. Prescribe treatment for diabetic ketoacidosis/diabetic coma.

Dr. Rajesh
76, Basent Vihar, Delhi
Regd. No. 2003/UCMS/642
Dated : 10-07-04

Sunil
24 yr/M
Regd. No. 1213

Δ   Diabetic Ketoacidosis

℞

Inj. Regular Insulin 1 ml vial.

Inj. Potassium chloride 500 mg vial.

Inj. Normal saline 500 ml vac.

Send 1 ml (40 U) regular insulin, 3 vials of potassium chloride (500 mg KCl in each vial) and 6 vacs of normal saline.

Inject insulin 0.2 U/Kg i/v stat followed by 0.1 U/kg/hr by slow i/v infusion. Give normal saline 1 litre/hour and add 20 mEq/hr potassium chloride (1 mEq = 75.5 mg) after 4 hours in the intravenous fluid.

Rajesh
2003/UCMS/642

---

8. Prescribe drug treatment for a patient of Renal Colic.

Dr. Rajesh
76, Basent Vihar, Delhi
Regd. No. 2003/UCMS/642
Dated : 10-07-04

Sunil
24 yr/M
Regd. No. 1213

Δ   Renal Colic

℞

Inj. Hyoscine butylbromide 1 ml (20 mg) amp.

Inj. Diclofenac sodium 3 ml amp. (1 ml = 25 mg)

Send two ampules of each drug.

Inject one ampoule of both drugs i/m stat and repeat if necessary.

Rajesh
2003/UCMS/642

9. Prescribe the drug treatment for a patient of cholera.

Dr. Rajesh
76, Basent Vihar, Delhi
Regd. No. 2003/UCMS/642
Dated : 10-07-04

Sunil
24 yr/M
Regd. No. 1213

Δ Cholera

℞

Oral Rehydration Salt

Tab. Doxycycline 100 mg.

Send such 10 tablets and two packets of ORS.

One tablet to be taken BD for 5 days and dissolve one packet of ORS in one litre water and take after every stool.

Rajesh
2003/UCMS/642

---

10. Prescribe the drug treatment for a pregnant female suffering from Tuberculosis.

Dr. Rajesh
76, Basent Vihar, Delhi
Regd. No. 2003/UCMS/642
Dated : 10-07-04

Sunil
26 yr/F
Regd. No. 1213

Δ Tuberculosis

℞

Tab. Isoniazid 300 mg
Tab. Rifampicin 600 mg
Tab. Pyrazinamide 1500 mg
Tab. Pyridoxine 10 mg

Send 180 tablets of Isoniazid, Rifampicin and Pyridoxine and 60 tablets of Pyrazinamide.

Take one tablet of Isoniazid, Rifampicin, Pyridoxine and Pyrazinamide OD per orally for 2 months followed by one tablet of Isoniazide, Rifampicm and Pyridoxine OD per orally for next 4 months.

Rajesh
2003/UCMS/642

---

11. Prescribe drug treatment for a hypertensive emergency.

Dr. Rajesh
76, Basent Vihar, Delhi
Regd. No. 2003/UCMS/642
Dated : 10-07-04

Sunil
24 yr/M
Regd. No. 1213

Δ   Hypertensive Emergency

℞

Inj. Sodium Nitroprusside 5 ml vial (1 ml = 10 mg)

Send such one vial.

Mix with 500 ml normal saline and give i/v infusion at a rate of 0.1 mg/min. till the B.P. is controlled.

Rajesh
2003/UCMS/642

---

12. Prescribe treatment for Anaphylactic shock.

Dr. Rajesh
76, Basent Vihar, Delhi
Regd. No. 2003/UCMS/642
Dated : 10-02-04

Sunil
24 yr/M
Regd. No. 1213

Δ   Anaphylactic Shock

℞

Inj. adrenaline hydrochloride 1 ml amp. (1 ml = 1 mg)

Send such one ampoule.

Half Ampule to be injected i/m stat.

Rajesh
2003/UCMS/642

13. Prescribe drug treatment for an obese middle aged diabetic

---

Dr. Rajesh
76, Basent Vihar, Delhi
Regd. No. 2003/UCMS/642
Dated : 10-07-04

Sunil
44 yr/M
Regd. No. 1213

   Δ Type II Diabetes Mellitus

Rx

    Tab. Metformin 500 mg

    Send such 14 tablets

    One tablet to be taken BD per orally for 7 days and review after 7 days.

               Rajesh
               2003/UCMS/642

---

14. Prescribe drug treatment for Trichomonial infection

Dr. Rajesh
76, Basent Vihar, Delhi
Regd. No. 2003/UCMS/642
Dated : 10-07-04

Sunil
24 yr/M
Regd. No. 1213

   Δ Trichomoniasis

Rx

    Tab. Metronidazole 400 mg.

    Send such 21 tablets

    Take one tablet TDS per orally for 7 days.

               Rajesh
               2003/UCMS/642

---

* **Note:** Alternative drugs are:

 1. Tinidazole 600 mg OD × 7 days

 2. Secnidazole 2 gm single oral dose

15. Prescribe for a patient having anemia with piles.

Dr. Rajesh
76, Basent Vihar, Delhi
Regd. No. 2003/UCMS/642
Dated : 10-07-04

Sunil
24 yr/M
Regd. No. 1213

Δ   Anemia with Piles.

℞

Tab. Ferrous Sulphate 200 mg

Phenol 5 ml

Almond Oil 95 ml

Send 90 tablets of ferrous sulphate and mix and make solution of phenol in almond oil and send such 5 ml.

5 ml of the solution to be injected in the piles and take one tablet of ferrous sulphate TDS per orally for one month.

Rajesh
2003/UCMS/642

---

16. Priscribe the drug treatment for a patient with hypovolemic shock.

Dr. Rajesh
76, Basent Vihar, Delhi
Regd. No. 2003/UCMS/642
Dated : 10-07-04

Sunil
24 yr/M
Regd. No. 1213

Δ Hypovolemic Shock

℞

Inj. Normal saline 500 ml vac.

Inj. Dopamine 2 ml amp. (1 ml = 80 mg)

Send two vac. of normal saline and two amp. of dopamine.

Add one ampoule of dopamine to one vac. of normal saline and give by slow i/v infusion at a rate of 2 mg/kg/min.

Rajesh
2003/UCMS/642

17. Prescribe the treatment for a patient suffering from infestation with pinworm.

Dr. Rajesh
76, Basent Vihar, Delhi
Regd. No. 2003/UCMS/642
Dated : 10-07-04

Sunil
24 yr/M
Regd. No. 1213

    Δ   Pinworm infestation

℞

        Tab. Albendazole 400 mg
        Send such one tablet.
        Take the tablet per orally at night.

                        Rajesh
                        2003/UCMS/642

---

18. Prescribe for a patient with Roundworm infestation.

Dr. Rajesh
76, Basent Vihar, Delhi
Regd. No. 2003/UCMS/642
Dated : 10-07-04

Sunil
24 yr/M
Regd. No. 1213

    Δ   Ascariasis

℞

        Tab. Albendazole 400 mg
        Send such one tablet
        Take the tablet per orally at night.

                        Rajesh
                        2003/UCMS/642

---

19. Prescribe the drug treatment for a patient suffering from amoebic colitis.

Dr. Rajesh
76, Basent Vihar, Delhi
Regd. No. 2003/UCMS/642
Dated : 10-07-04

Sunil
24 yr/M
Regd. No. 1213

Δ   Ameobic Colitis

℞

Tab. Metronidazole 400 mg.

Tab. Diloxanide furoate 500 mg

Tab. Hyoscine butylbromide 10 mg

Send 15 tablets of Metronidazole, 30 tablets of diloxanide furoate and 4 tablets of hyoscine butyl bromide.

Take one tablet of Metronidazole and diloxanide furoate TDS per orally for five days and continue diloxanide for 5 more days. Take tab. Hyoscine butylbromide whenever there is colicky pain in abdomen.

Rajesh
2003/UCMS/642

20. Prescribe drug treatment for a patient suffering from hookworm infestation.

Dr. Rajesh
76, Basent Vihar, Delhi
Regd. No. 2003/UCMS/642
Dated : 10-07-04

Sunil
24 yr/M
Regd. No. 1213

Δ   Ancylostomiasis

℞

Tab. Albendazole 400 mg

Tab. Ferrous sulphate 200 mg

Send one tablet of albendazole and 90 tablets of ferrous sulphate.

Take tablet of albendazole per orally at night and take one tablet of ferrous sulphate TDS per orally for one month.

Rajesh
2003/UCMS/642

21. Prescribe drug treatment for a patient suffering from peptic ulcer.

Dr. Rajesh
76, Basent Vihar, Delhi
Regd. No. 2003/UCMS/642
Dated : 10-07-04

Sunil
24 yr/M
Regd. No. 1213

Δ   Peptic Ulcer

℞

        Tab. Omeprazole 20 mg

        Send such 28 tablets

        One tablet to be taken OD per orally for 4 weeks.

          Rajesh
          2003/UCMS/642

---

22. Prescribe treatment for acute attack of Myocardial infarction.

Dr. Rajesh
76, Basent Vihar, Delhi
Regd. No. 2003/UCMS/642
Dated : 10-07-04

Sunil
24 yr/M
Regd. No. 1213

Δ   Acute attack of Myocardial Infarction

℞

        Inj. Morphine 1 ml vial (1 ml = 10 mg)

        Inj. streptokinase 7.5 lac I.U. vial

        Tab. Aspirin 75 mg

        Send one vial each of morphine and streptokinase and 30 tablets of aspirin.

        Inject morphine sulphate half vial i/v, followed by another injection after 30 minutes, if pain persists. Give oxygen inhalation at a rate of 4 L/minute. Give slow i/v injection of Streptokinase 7.5 lac I.U. over 1 hr and give tablet aspirin OD per orally for lifelong.

          Rajesh
          2003/UCMS/642

23. Prescribe for a patient of angina during and in between attacks.

Dr. Rajesh
76, Basent Vihar, Delhi
Regd. No. 2003/UCMS/642
Dated : 10-07-04

Sunil
24 yr/M
Regd. No. 1213

Δ   Angina pectoris

℞

Tab. Glyceryltrinitrate 0.5 mg

Tab. Isosorbide dinitrate 10 mg

Send one tablet of Glyceryltrinitrate and seven tablets of Isosorbide dinitrate.

Take tablet of GTN sublingually and one tablet of Isosorbide dinitrate OD per orally for 7 days and review after 7 days.

Rajesh
2003/UCMS/642

---

24. Prescribe for a patient of acute asthma with upper respiratory tract Infector.

Dr. Rajesh
76, Basent Vihar, Delhi
Regd. No. 2003/UCMS/642
Dated : 10-07-04

Sunil
24 yr/M
Regd. No. 1213

Δ   Acute Asthma with Upper Respiratory Tract Infection.

℞

Cap. Amoxycillin 500 mg

Salbutamol nebulization solution - 1 ml vial (1 ml = 5 mg)

Send 15 capsules of Amoxycillin and two vials of salbutamol nebulization solution

Nebulize with 1 ml solution intermittently and take one capsule TDS per orally for 5 days.

Rajesh
2003/UCMS/642

25. Prescribe for a patient suffering from Lobar Pheumonia.

Dr. Rajesh
76, Basent Vihar, Delhi
Regd. No. 2003/UCMS/642
Dated : 10-07-04

Sunil
24 yr/M
Regd. No. 1213

Δ   Lobar Pneumonia

℞

Tab. Erythromycin 50 mg

Tab. Paracetamol 500 mg

Send 28 tablets of erythromycin and 9 tablets of paracetamol.

Take one tablet of erythromycin QID per orally for 7 days and one tablet of paracetamol TDS per orally for 3 days.

Rajesh
2004/UCMS/642

---

26. Prescribe treatment for a patient suffering from severe hypertension.

Dr. Rajesh
76, Basent Vihar, Delhi
Regd. No. 2003/UCMS/642
Dated : 10-07-04

Sunil
24 yr/M
Regd. No. 1213

Δ   Severe hypertension

℞

Tab. Lisinopril 5 mg

Tab. Atenolol 50 mg

Tab. Hydrochlorthiazide 12.5 mg

Send such 7 tablets of each drug.

Take one tablet of each drug OD per orally for 7 days and review after 7 days.

Rajesh
2003/UCMS/642

27. Prescribe the drug treatment for Left ventricular failure.

Dr. Rajesh
76, Basent Vihar, Delhi
Regd. No. 2003/UCMS/642

Sunil
24 yr/M
Regd. No. 1213

    Δ   Acute Left ventricular failure.

℞

        Inj. Furosemide 2 ml amp. (1 ml = 10 mg)

        Inj. Morphine 1 ml amp. (1 ml = 10 mg)

        Send 2 ampules of furosemide and 1 amp. of morphine.

        Give O_2 inhalation at 4L/min. and inject furosemide 2 ampules i/v stat and inject morphine one ampoule i/v.

                               Rajesh
                                 2003/UCMS/642

---

28. Prescribe treatment for a patient suffering from Kala Azar.

Dr. Rajesh
76, Basent Vihar, Delhi
Regd. No. 2003/UCMS/642
Dated : 10-07-04

Sunil
24 yr/M
Regd. No. 1213

    Δ   Leishmaniasis

℞

        Inj. Sodium stibogluconate 30 ml vial (1 ml = 100 mg)

        Send such 10 vials.

        (Inject half vial i/m daily for 20 days.)

                                 Rajesh
                                 2003/UCMS/642

29. Prescribe treatment for a patient suffering from Malasia.

Dr. Rajesh
76, Basent Vihar, Delhi
Regd. No. 2003/UCMS/642
Dated : 10-07-04

Sunil
24 yr/M
Regd. No. 1213

Δ   Malaria

℞

Tab. Chloroquine (150 mg base)

Tab. Primaquine 15 mg

Send 10 tablets of Chloroquine and 14 tablets of primaquine.

Take 4 tablets of Chloroquine P.O. stat followed by 2 tablets after 8 hours and then two tablets daily for next 2 days. Take tablet primaquine P.O. once daily for 14 days.

Rajesh
2003/UCMS/642

NOTES

NOTES

PART-V
CLINICAL CASES

CLINICAL CASES

CASE-1

Saurabh, 25 year old male is suffering from fever and was given Chloramphenicol 500 mg QID. Fever came down after two days but on 9th day he developed sore throat and mild fever. On heamatological examination, the findings are

RBC - 4 million/mm^3
WBC - 2200/mm^3
Neutrophil - 40%

Q. 1. What is the cause of sore throat & fever that developed on 9th day?

Ans. Chloramphenicol is a drug which is known to cause bone marrow depression leading to agranulocytosis. As the blood picture also confirms the depressed bone marrow function, the most likely cause of the these symptoms seems to be the decreased WBC level in blood.

Q. 2. How will you manage this case?

Ans. Chloramphenicol should be stopped immediately and other antibiotics like ciprofloxacin, amoxycillin or cephalosporins should be given Cotrimoxazole is also contraindicated, as it can also cause bone marrow depression.

CASE-2

A 50 year old patient Sudhir Kumar presented to emergency department of Guru Teg Bahadur Hospital at 2 a.m. with complaints of severe breathlessness and orthophoea. On Examination, there was severe edema of feet and coarse hissing rales were heard all over the chest. He was given some medication and in the morning, he was comfortable and passed 3 litres of unine. Serum electrolyte levels were as follows

Na$^+$ - 150 mEq/L
K$^+$ - 20 mEq/L
Cl$^-$ - 155 mEq/L

Q. 1. What is the possible diagnosis of the patient?

Ans. Most probably the patient may be suffering from acute pulmonary edema as indicated by symptoms of breathlessness and orthopnoea along with examination findings of edema feet and coarse crepitations in chest. It may be due to acute left ventricular failure.

Q. 2. What are the that drugs may have been given at night?

Ans. Some diuretics like furosemide may have been given to relieve the congestive symptoms. Relief of the symptoms of the patient along with passage of large amount of urine points towards the use of a diuretic.

Q. 3. What others drugs should be used in this case?

Ans. The other drug that should be used along with oxygen inhalation is morphine. It relieves pain, decongests the lungs by shifting blood from pulmonary to systemic circulation and also allays anxiety.

CASE-3

Sunita, 40 year old female had spells of dizziners and palpitations for 6 months. These episodes occurred around 6 to 6.30 p.m. and were relieved by a glass of milk. There was no loss of consciousness.

She also reported a history of diabetes mellitus since 4 years. She was following a strict dietary control and her blood sugar was satisfactorily controlled on glibenclamide 5 mg before breakfast and 2.5 mg before dinner. 6 months ago, she also developed arthritis and was put on variable dose of aspirin.

Her Fasting Blood glucose was found to be 80 mg% and the X-Ray of her hands revealed a soft tissue swelling of metacarpophalyngeal joints.

Q. 1. What is the cause of the patient's symptoms?

Ans. The symptoms are due to hypoglycemia. The cause of hypoglycemia seems to be aspirin. Aspirin causes increased utilization of glucose in the body, particularly in diabetic. Also aspirin displaces glibenclamide from plasma protein binding sites. Both of these actions result in hypoglycemia.

Q. 2. What measures should be taken in this case?

Ans. First of all, the patient must be educated not to go hungry or miss a meal. She should keep glucose or biscuit with her, so that if hypoglycemia is suspected, the dangerous consequences can be avoided. The dose of glibenclamide should be reduced or alternative NSAIDS to aspirin like ibuprofen can be used.

CASE-4

Manohar, 28 years old male presented to the hospital with complaints of headache, fever, with chills off and on for the last 8 days. On examination he was pale. His temperature was 103° F with a pulse rate of 122/min. Spleen was enlarged and palpable, 2 fingers below costal margin.

Q. 1. What is the most likely diagnosis?

Ans. Most probably, Manohar is suffering from malasia.

Q. 2. How will you manage this patient?

Ans. We will take the blood sample of the patient when the fever is at a peak and send it for peripheral smear examination for malarial parasite, and the patient will be given paracetamol 500 mg and cold sponging for the fever. Chloroquine will also be started Chloroquine will be given at a dose of 600 mg base stat, then 300 mg after 8 hours followed by 300 mg daily for the next two days. If on peripheral smear, Plasmodium falciparum is seen, this treatment is satisfactory but if Plasmodium vivax is seen, this treatment will be followed by primaquine 15 mg daily for 2 weeks.

Q. 3. What other drugs are used to treat this condition?

Ans. Other drugs are mefloquine, quinine, phyrimethamine, halofantrine, artemisin derivatives etc.

CASE-5

Raju, 15 years old male with severe vomiting and diarrhoea was given the following treatment.

Inj metoclopramide 10 mg i.v. stat
Tab. metoclopramide 10 mg tds
Tab. ciprofloxacin 500 mg BD
Tab. loperamide 4 mg BD

About 30 min following treatment, the boy developed upward rolling of eyes and the neck was stretched to one side. the boy was shifted to the emergency.

Q. 1. What is the cause of secondary symptoms after the treatment?

Ans. The most likely cause of the secondary symptoms is the extra phyramidal side effect of metoclopramide (known as perinorm, reaction). By blocking dopamine receptors, metoclopramide may cause dystonias.

Q. 2. How will you manage such a case?

Ans. After stabilizing the patient and maintaining, patency of airways, breathing and circulation, the patient should be prescribed some central anticholinergic drug like trihexyphenidyl.

Q. 3. Comment on the treatments given to patient.

Ans. Loperamide is not recommended in infective diarrhea, so the treatment is not rational.

CASE-6

An asthmatic pregnant female at term was admitted to labour room. She showed signs of impending attack of asthma for which she was given salbutamol. She showed diminished labour pains.

Q. 1. What is the cause of decreased labour pains?

Ans. Salbutamol by its β-agonistic action may cause decreased contractility of uterus leading to decreased labour pains.

Q. 2. How should she have been managed?

Ans. She should be given aminophylline by slow i/v infusion and ipratropium bromide may also be used.

CASE-7

Sonali Mahajan is a 52 year old female who presented to the OPD for routine opthalmic examination. Her visual activity without correction was 1/6 (Right eye) and 1/60 (left eye). Tonometry measured an intraocular pressure of 36 mm hg in both eyes. Opthalmoscopy revealed physiologic cupping of the optic disc and visual field defects. Both pupils were normal and gonioscopy indicated that anterior chamber angles were normal and there were no sign of cataract formation.

Q. 1. What is the probable diagnosis?

Ans. Primary open angle glaucoma.

Q. 2. Write the treatment to be given to Sonali.

Ans.1. β Adrenergic blockers: Timolol 0.25% drops BD, Betaxolol 0.5% drops BD

2. Miotics : Pilocarpine 0.5% QID.
   Physostigmine 0.1%

3. α Adrenergic agonists : Adrenaline
   Apraclonidine
   Brimonidine
   Dipivefrine

4. Carbonic anhydrase inhibitors :
   Acetazolamide   0.25 g orally BD
   Dorzolamide   2% drops TDS

5. Prostaglandins: Latanoprost (PG_2F_α)

Q. 3. Enumerate the adverse effects of topical miotics and B blockers.

Miotics

1. Constriction of pupil leads to diminution of vision in dim light.
2. May induce myopia in young patients.
3. Headache & brow pain due to spasm of iris & ciliary muscles.
4. Fluctuations in i.o.t. may occur.

β-blockers

1. Stinging, burning and redness in eye
2. Dryness of eyes
3. Allergic Blepharoconjuctivitis
4. Corneal hypoasthesia
5. Blurred vision

CASE-8

Meena a 9 yr old girl, is reported by her teacher to have 3-4 episodes of staring daily. Each spell lasts about 5-10 seconds. there are no convulsive movements although her eyelids appear to flutter during the episodes. She is fully alert afterwards. An EEG shows 3/ second spike-wave activity. No positive findings are found on neurological examination.

Q. 1. Write the probable diagnosis.

Ans. Petil Mal Epilepsy (Absence seizures)

Q. 2. What should be the treatment?

Ans. Valproate : 15-30 mg/kg/day.
    or
    Ethosuximide 20-30 mg/kg/day.
    Valproate is more commonly used because it also prevents kindling and emergence of GTCS. Otherwise both are equally efficacious.

Q. 3. What are the major side effects of valproate therapy?

Ans. 1. Alopecia
2. Curling of hair
3. Anorexia
4. Vomiting
5. Drowsiness

CASE-9

An eighteen year old female Shehnaz Khan was brought to the accident and emergency ward of GTB Hospital in an unconscious state by her relatives. The mother told the attending doctor that her daughter was well is the morning. Today in the morning her CBSE results were declared and she had failed in the examination for the third time. She went to the local market and then to her room. After sometime when her mother entered the rooms, she found Shehnaz unconscious with fluid drooling out from her mouth. An empty bottle was found lying by her side.

Upon arrival the patient was salivating profusely. Her extremities were cold; BP 90/60 hg. Pulse 68/mn, regular, RR 30/min. There was no evidence of trauma. Both pupils were constricted and did not respond to light. Extremities showed occasional subcutaneous muscle fasciculations at the time of admission which disappeared during examination; however the muscles were flaccid and breathing was shallow. Neurological examination revealed coma with no response to painful stimuli. Chest examination revealed moderate wheezing. No other abnormality was found.

Q. 1. What is the most likely cause of the patient's condition?

Ans. Organophosphate poisoning.

Q. 2. What is the management of the patient?

Ans. 1. Termination of further exposure to poison by gastric lavage.

2. Mantain patent airway, positive pressure respiration

3. Maintain BP, hydration

4. Specific antidotes:-

(a) Atropine 2 mg iv repeated every 10 min till pupils dilate (maximum 200 mg).

(b) Cholinesterase reactivators : Pralidoxime 1-2g iv slowly. 20-40 mg/kg in children.

Q. 3. Identify the receptors involved for

(a) excessive salivation, bradycardia and miosis

(b) Fasciculation in the muscle and breathing difficulties.

Ans:

CASE-10

5 year old child Guddu, was brought to the hospital with complaint of recurrent vomiting. He was given 10 mg perinorm (metoclopramide) as anti-emetic. The child became drowsy and then developed muscle dystonia and myoclonus.

Questions

1. Why did the child developed there symptoms?

Ans. The child has developed 'Perinorm reaction' i.e. the extrapyramidal side effects of metoclopramide. Metoclopramide is a D_2 receptor blocker and the blockade of dopaminergic receptors in the central nervous system results in extrapyramidal symptoms as seen in this case.

2. What is the mechanism of action of meteclopramide?

Ans. Metoclopramide acts by various mechanisms. These are

(a) D_2 receptor blockade in G.I.T. resulting in increased gastric emptying and increased tone of Lower Esophageal Sphinctor.

(b) D_2 receptor blockade at Chemoreceptor Trigger Zone (CTZ).

(c) Enhanced Ach release from myenteric plexus in G.I.T.

(d) At high doses, it blocks $5HT_3$ receptors in G.I.T. and C.T.Z.

3. What should be the right prescription and why?

Ans. Perinorm should not be prescribed to the child because children are more susceptible to the extrapyramidal side effects of the drug. Instead, domperidone should be given which does not cross blood brain barrier and thus no extrapyramidal side effects are produced.

CASE-11

Mr. Prashant, 28 years old man was brought to hospital with symptoms of vomiting, headache, epigastric pain, difficulty in breathing and blurring of vision. These symptoms started after drinking alcohol. On examination, there is decreased heart rate and blood pressure and acidosis is confirmed on arterial blood gas analysis.

Q. 1. What is the possible cause of the signs & symptoms of the patient?

Q. 2. How should the patient be treated?

Ans.

1. The likely cause in this case is 'methyl alcohol poisoning'. The patient may have drunk alcohol in which methanol (methyl alcohol) has been mixed. Methyl alcohol is metabolized to formaldehyde & finally to formic acid by alcohol dehydrogenase and aldehyde dehydrogenase respectively.

$$\text{Methyl Alcohol} \xrightarrow[\text{dehydrogenase}]{\text{Alcohol}} \text{Formaldehyde}$$
$$(\text{CH}_3\text{OH}) \qquad\qquad\qquad (\text{HCHO})$$

$$\xrightarrow[\text{dehydrogenase}]{\text{Aldehyde}} \text{Formic Acid}$$
$$\qquad\qquad (\text{HCOOH})$$

Blood level of 750 mg/dl of methanol is associated with severe poisoning. Above signs and symptoms are mainly due to formic acid. Acidosis is prominent and retinal damage is a specific toxicity of formic acid resulting in blurring of vision & finally blindness.

2. Treatment of methyl alcohol poisoning is done as follows.

1. Eyes should be protected from light and patient should be kept in a quiet and dark room.

2. Gastric lavage should be done with sodium bicarbonate to remove unabsorbed methyl alcohol.

PART-VI
COMMENTS

1. *Statement:* A patient of Leukemia on 6-mercaptopurine therapy was given allopurinol for his high serum uric acid levels.

Comment: The dose of 6-mercaptopurine (6-MP) should be reduced to one third, because allopurinol inhibits the degradation of 6-MP. It is metabolised by xanthine oxidase and allopurinol is an inhibitor of this enzyme. Therefore it is necessary to reduce the dose of 6-MP in order to avoid its toxic effects.

2. *Statement:* A patient of parkinsonism on L-DOPA therapy alone was given pyridoxine.

Comment: Pyridoxine abolishes the therapeutic effect of L-DOPA, therefore it should not be given along with L-DOPA. In Parkinsonism, there is an imbalance between dopamine and acetylcholine levels in the brain. Dopamine levels are decreased whereas acetylcholine levels are relatively increased. L-DOPA crosses the Blood Brain Barrier (BBB) and undergoes decarboxylation to get converted to dopamine. It is also decarboxylated in the peripheral tissues and the dopamine formed is not able to cross BBB. Excess of dopamine in the periphery is responsible for its adverse effects. The little amount of L-DOPA (~1-2 %) that remains is able to cross BBB and is responsible for the therapeutic effect. Pyridoxine on the other hand enhances the peripheral decarboxylation of l-DOPA to dopamine, because it is a cofactor for the enzyme dopa-decarboxylase. Thus less of L-DOPA is available to cross BBB.

3. *Statement:* Sodium bicarbonate is prescribed to a patient of urinary tract infection who is being treated with nitrofurantoin.

Comment: Sodium bicarbonate is an alkali and causes the alkalinization of urine. Nitrofurantoin is more effective at an acidic pH of urine. Therefore sodium bicarbonate should not be given along with nitrofurantoin as it will cause blunting of the effect of nitrofurantoin.

4. *Statement:* A patient of congestive heart failure is receiving digoxin and thiazide.

Comment: Digoxin and thiazides should not be given together. This is because thiazide has a tendency to cause hypokalemia which accentuates the toxicity of digoxin. Thus, the patient will be at more risk of digoxin-induced arrythmias. Either potassium supplements should be added or thiazide should be replaced by potassium sparing diuretics in this patient.

Statement 5: A patient of gout receiving Probenecid is given thiazide for hypertension.

Comment: This combination is not rational because probenecid and thiazide both decrease each other's effect. Thiazide is secreted in the tubular fluid and reaches its site of action (distal tubules) Probenecid competes with thiazide secretion and thereby decreases its concentration at the site of action resulting in decreased therapeutic effect. On the other hand, thiazide causes hyperuricemia, thus opposing the uricosuric effect of probenecid. To prevent this interaction, thiazides should be replaced by other anti hypertensive drugs like beta blockers or ACE inhibitors.

Statement 6: A female taking oral contraceptives acquired tuberculosis and was prescribed a regimen containing rifampicin and isoniazide.

Comment: Rifampicin is a microsomal enzyme inducer leading to enhanced metabolism of many drugs including oral contraceptives. So, rifampicin can cause contraception failure. Patient should switch over to an oral contraceptive pill containing higher concentration of estrogen (50 mg instead of 30 mg) Rifampicin should not be replaced as it is most effective anti tubercular drug.

Statement 7: A patient of pernicious anaemia is prescribed Tab Cyanocobalamin 10 mg thrice a day.

Comment: Pernicious anemia is due to incomplete absorption of vitamin B_{12} from gastrointestinal tract because of deficiency of intrinsic factor. Oral cyanocobalamin (B_{12}) will not be absorbed in such a situation. Therefore treatment of pernicious anemia should be with parental (either intramuscular or subcutaneous) vitamin B_{12}. The dose of vitamin B_{12} is 30-100 mg/day for first 10 days followed by 100 mg weekly and then 100 mg monthly for life.

Statement 8: A patient of deep vein thrombosis on acenocoumarin received aspirin for headache.

Comment: Aspirin should not be given to a patient taking anticoagulants. Acenocoumarin is an oral anticoagulant and aspirin increases the risk of bleeding especially from gastrointestinal tract because:-

  i) It inhibits platelet aggregation
  ii) High dose of aspirin decreases serum prothrombin.
  iii) It also displaces oral anticoagulants from plasma protein binding sites; thus increasing their levels in the blood.

Therefore, in this case either the dose of acenocoumarin should be reduced or aspirin should be replaced by ibuprofen.

Statement 9. A patient of mania receiving lithium developed pulmonary edema for which furosemide was prescribed.

Comment: Furosemide should not be given to this patient. Diuretics like furosemide and thiazides cause reabsorption of Li^+ and thus may cause lithium toxicity. This is because diuretics cause excessive Na^+ loss which results in more Na^+ reabsorption by kidneys in order to maintain Na^+ levels in blood. Kidneys handle Li^+ in the same way as Na^+, therefore Li^+ is also reabsorbed. In order to avoid this lithium toxicity, the dose of lithium should be decreased and serum levels should be carefully monitored and kept between 0.5 - 0.8 mEq/L for maintenance therapy and 0.8 - 1.1 mEq/L for treatment of acute mania.

Statement 10: A patient of whooping cough on tetracycline therapy developed pain abdomen on second day of therapy, for which aluminium hydroxide was prescribed.

Comment: Aluminium hydroxide decreases the absorption of tetracycline by raising the gastric pH and by forming non-absorbable complexes with tetracycline, so the two drugs should be given at a gap of atleast 2 hours.

Statement 11. A patient of pulmonary edema on furosemide developed chest infection for which gentamycin was prescribed.

Comment: This is not a rationale combination as both high ceiling diuretics (e.g. furosemide) and

aminoglycosides (like gentamycin) cause ototoxicity. Therefore in this case, some other antibiotic like cephalosporins should be prescribed for chest infection.

Statement 12: A patient of tuberculosis on streptomycin therapy has to undergo surgery. Vecuronium is used as the skeletal muscle relaxant.

Comment: This combination is dangerous because it may cause prolonged apnoea. Aminoglycosides (streptomycin in this case) augment the action of competitive neuromuscular blockers like vecuronium by decreasing ach release from pre junctional nerve endings. So, the dose of vecuronium should be decreased.

Statement 13: A patient on warfarin therapy developed urinary tract infection for which cefoperazone was prescribed.

Comment: The chances of bleeding will increase if cefoperazone is given along with oral anti-coagulants because cefoperazone causes hypoprothrombinemia. So, either the dose of warfarin should be reduced or a different antibiotic like nor floxacin should be prescribed.

Statement 14: A patient on amphetamine therapy was given sodium bicarbonate.

Comment: Amphetamine is a basic drug, so it is ionized more at acidic ph. which results in its rapid excretion. Sodium bicarbonate causes alkalinization and thus causes reabsorption or amphetamine. This decreased excretion predisposes to toxicity.

Statement 15: A patient of status asthmaticus was prescribed ephedrine 100 mg tds.

Comment: Ephedrine causes slowly developing bronchodilation, so it is not suitable for emergency conditions like status asthmaticus where immediate bronchodilation is required. It is thus more suitable for mild or moderate chronic bronchial asthma. The patient in this case, should have been managed rigorously with intravenous hydrocortisone, oxygen inhalation and nebulized salbutamol.

Statement 16: Patient having diarrhoea was given metronidazole 400 mg TDS. At night, he developed flushing, throbbing headache, vomiting and confusion.

Comment: The symptoms of the patient are suggestive of aldehyde syndrome (Disulfiram like reaction). The patient might have taken alcohol at night. Metronidazole inhibits the enzyme aldehyde dehydro-genase which results in increased concentration of aldehydes in the blood that is responsible for above symptoms.

$$CH_3CH_2OH \xrightarrow[\text{dehydrogenase}]{\text{Alcohol}} CH_3CHO$$
(Ethyl Alcohol) (Acetaldehyde)

$$\xrightarrow[\text{dehydrogenase}]{\text{Aldehyde}} CH_3COOH$$
(Acetic acid)

The patient must be instructed to avoid alcohol if he is prescribed metronidazole.

Statement 17: A patient for whom succinylcholine was used as skeletal muscle relaxant was given neostigmine post operatively.

Comment: Neostigmime is a cholinesterase inhibitor which is used to reverse the action of competitive skeletal muscle relaxants like vecuronium. The effect of succinylcholine will not be reversed as it is a non-competitive or depolarizing type of neuromuscular blocker. On the contrary, the blocking action of succinyl-choline at neuromuscular junction is potentiated by neostigmine. Furthermore, the duration of action of Sch is very short and the action terminates by itself. Therefore, neostigmine should not be prescribed.

Statement 18: A patient of pheochromocytoma was given β-Blocker to control hypertension.

Comment: β-Blockers taken alone by a patient of pheochromocytoma will result in severe rise of blood pressure. In pheochromocytoma, there are excess of catecholamines in the blood. If β-receptors are blocked, they will act only on α-receptors. Therefore severe vasoconstriction occurs due to unopposed α-action resulting in hypertensive crisis. Due to this reason, β-Blockers should be given only after blocking the α-action.

Statement 19: A patient of angina was prescribed aspirin 500 mg per day for prophylaxis.

Comment: Low dose of aspirin (160-325 mg) inhibits cyclooxygenase enzyme present in platelets. Platelets produce thromboxane A$_2$ (TXA$_2$), which has proaggregatory properties. Due to decreased formation of TXA$_2$ by aspirin treatment, it produces antiplatelet action. On the other hand, high dose of aspirin inhibits not only the cycloxygenase present in platelets but also that in the endothelium. The inhibition of endothelial cycloxygenase decreases the production of prostacyclins (PGI$_2$), which itself has

anti-aggregatory properties. Therefore low dose of aspirin (160-325 mg) should be used for antiplatelet action.

Statement 20: A patient of gout developed angina for which aspirin 160 mg/day was prescribed

Comment: Aspirin at low doses inhibits uric acid excretion thus aggravating gout. But at higher doses, aspirin acts as a uricosuric agent. Since at high doses antiplatelet action of aspirin is lost, it is not recommended in a patient of angina with gout. Alternative antiplatelet drugs like clopidogrel should be used in such a case.

Statement 21: A female with 34 week pregnancy was given ergometrine for induction of labour.

Comment: Ergometrine causes contraction of all segments of uterus which precipitates fetal distress as the presenting part is compressed against the contracted cervix. For induction of labour, fundus and upper uterine segment should be contracted with relaxation of lower uterine segment. Oxytocin has this property of mimicking the physiological contraction of uterus. Therefore, Oxytocin should have been used instead of ergometrine for induction of labour.

Statement 22: A patient diagnosed to be suffering from pernicious anemia is given folic acid.

Comment: Pernicious anemia is due to deficiency of intrinsic factor as a result of formation of autoantibodies against gastric parietal cells. Deficiency of intrinsic factor leads to decreased vitamin B$_{12}$ absorption and consequently megaloblastic anemia vitamin. B$_{12}$ performs two main functions.

1. It converts methyl tetrahydrofolic acid (Methyl-THFA) to THFA; which is essential for one carbon unit transfer and DNA synthesis.

2. It results in conversion of homocysteine to methionine which is used in formation of myelin sheath.

When folic acid is given to a patient of pernicious anemia, the small amount of vitamin B$_{12}$ present in the body is utilized for the conversion of methyl THFA to THFA and thus DNA is formed and blood cells are matured leading to correction of blood picture. But, there is no B$_{12}$ left to form methionine. As a result myelin sheath is not formed and neurological deficits (eg. subacute combined degeneration of spinal Cord) are aggravated.

Therefore, folic acid should be given in combination with vitamin B_{12} and not alone, in such a patient.

Statement 23: A 5 month old child suffering from upper respiratory tract infection was given tetracyclines.

Comment: This prescription is not rationale since tetracycline causes dentition and bone defects in children. It causes brown discolouration of teeth and deposits in the bone. It has chelating properties so it forms a complex with calcium present in the bone. The child should have been prescribed any other antibiotic like cotrimoxazole.

Statement 24: A patient of epilepsy on phenytoin treatment has Hb level of 4.5 gm% and was prescribed iron for this.

Comment: Patient may have developed anemia as a result of adverse effect of phenytoin. Phenytoin causes decreased absorption of folic acid resulting in megaloblastic anemia. Iron will not cure this condition. Therefore, the type of anemia should be tested by hematological examination and if found to be megaloblastic, folic acid should be prescribed.

NOTES

NOTES

NOTES